The Best of the Stroke Connection

Compiled by Pat Kasell
Courage Stroke Network

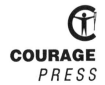

COURAGE
PRESS

Golden Valley, Minnesota

Publisher's Note

Where possible, permission has been received from each of the authors to publish their articles. Every attempt was made to contact the authors. To all of the writers we express our genuine appreciation and gratitude, for without them there would be no book.

The Best of the Stroke Connection

ISBN 0-9622455-3-4

Manufactured in the United States of America

Published by Courage Press, 3915 Golden Valley Road, Golden Valley, Minnesota 55422 U.S.A.

Dedication

To Justin Karon
whose persistent sensitivity
to stroke survivors
led to the birth of
the Courage Stroke Network

from the Stroke Connection June 1983

A 4th of July Victory

by Helen Rathje, Annandale, Minnesota

To be in Annandale for the big 4th of July celebration is to experience a memorable day—for those who just love to eat barbecued pork chops while listening to the screams from the direction of the thrill rides and the "oohs" and "aahs" of those watching for fireworks; for those who just like to sit around in the park and visit with friends; and for those who gather early, waiting for the start of the big parade.

I would like to tell you what it meant to someone whom I know very well. It was during the winter of '79 and '80 that this man began to train two of his favorite Belgian horses for the parade that July. But suddenly in mid-April he was stricken with complete paralysis of the left side of his body. The doctor diagnosed it as a stroke. Many long, painful months followed, along with major surgery in June. Hope was almost abandoned within the heart of this man and anyone else who was personally acquainted with him. After several months, he was discharged from the hospital. Arrangements were made for him to spend each day at a rest home in an environment of elderly people who had no hope of ever returning to their homes. Gradually he progressed from the bed to a wheelchair, then to a four-pronged cane, to a lighter cane and finally to no cane at all. Slowly he learned to walk again—to once again drive the car. He was able to have coffee with the guys at the restaurant and to return to some of the everyday activities of life that everyone takes so much for granted. He was able to return to church to worship and to thank everyone for their prayers and concern.

Eventually he was able to remain at home alone during the day, but spent many months making daily trips to the hospital for therapy. In spite of all the obstacles, he never gave up hope of being able to drive those horses. One would find him in the garage sitting on a chair, with harness lines attached to the vise on the workbench, practicing and strengthening the muscles of his left arm and hand.

Day after day he would sit in his favorite rocking chair and stare into space wondering and planning how he could accomplish his dream. During these months one of his sons and his grandsons cared for his horses daily, but the time came when a decision had to be made and he thought he would sell them. But this was not to be. An interested daughter-in-law, who herself loves horses, and his son said, "Dad, we'll help you if you want to drive them in the parade." The wagon was painted, the new harness that had hung in the garage for two years was fitted and the new task began. The horses were trained well enough to be brought into town. They crossed the railroad track—which can be very "iffy" with horses, so I am told. Every day he would watch the clock waiting for the time when everyone would again be free to help him. A step was made so he could get up in the box of the wagon. He was not able to harness the horses himself or to attend to the details so necessary to good horsemanship, but he had the strength to drive.

Finally, the big day came. The horses were groomed, harnessed and hitched. Even his granddaughter and pet dog were ready to ride. Perhaps you didn't even notice their unit in the parade. Perhaps you are one of the many who would rather water ski, fish, hunt, bowl or whatever. Perhaps you do not care for horses at all. But to one who loves horses, he accomplished what many people thought would never happen. He was able to drive his horses in the parade! The parade of a lifetime for him! Why am I writing this letter? How do I know so much about that day? He is my husband and I am thankful to everyone who helped to make this dream become a reality.

from the Stroke Connection January/February 1987

A Daughter's View of Stroke

by Krista Lee, St. Louis Park, Minnesota

I t has been five years since my mother had her stroke. My twin sister and I were just beginning our junior years at the University of Minnesota, each of us very involved with sorority life. My brother was a sophomore at St. Louis Park Senior High and involved with jazz band.

The night my mother was taken to the hospital was the longest night of our lives. The days and weeks that followed would become complicated by a situation that was out of our control. Slowly, the realization of the seriousness of my mother's stroke and the prognosis whirled us through a maze of emotions and actions.

I went through the normal stages of a traumatic experience: fear, worry, numbness, resentment and guilt. The unending hope makes all these other feelings so bittersweet. It was hard for me to deal with feelings that I had never experienced with such intensity before in my life. At first, I worried about my mother's immediate condition and prayed she would live because thinking about the future and the changes that would be inevitable was too overwhelming.

In a way, most of us tried to ignore the future. I tried to "wake up" from the whole nightmare. Sometimes, because I lived on campus and not in the family home, I could pretend that things were normal at home. I could block it all out for a while. But somehow there always was a little pang of worry in the back of my mind. I worried not only for my mother, but for my father and brother. They lived with the pain and agony every day. My sister and I could escape, but they couldn't. I often wonder if my father felt trapped in those first few months—like a caged animal that has no real control over what is going to happen. Dad had no choice in the matter—he merely had to survive every day and somehow support his wife in the hospital. These things bothered me as much as my mother lying in the

3

hospital. Would we all come through this without scars? Could we possibly survive and somehow not be changed? Five years later I know that it is impossible to come through an experience like this and not be changed.

My mother was in the hospital for nearly two months. The first month, she suffered severe pressure on the front part of her brain which resulted in incoherency and almost childlike behavior. My sister Kari and I visited every Tuesday and Thursday for a good portion of the day. I remember resenting the time I spent with my mother because I would rather have been laughing with my friends at school than sitting in a hospital room. One afternoon Kari and I were with my mother. She was doing badly that day and I remember her yelling out for strangers. Feeling helpless and quite embarrassed that my mother had lost that much control, the two of us burst into nervous giggles and spent the rest of the day trying to quiet her.

Sometimes I would forget she was sick and expect her to act the way she used to. When she wouldn't eat I had to keep myself from yelling at her. It was extremely difficult for a grown child to see her mother helpless and incapacitated. The role of caregiver was reversed and the natural child in all of us resents that reversal very deeply. The loss was deep because, in a way, I had lost my mother, yet she still lived. She wasn't the same and never would be quite the same again. She would never be able to hug me with both of her arms again; she wouldn't be able to take care of me because she was trying to heal herself. I felt very cheated. Instead of trying to understand her ordeal, I pulled away and tried to distance myself from the whole situation.

My mother came home from the hospital in time for Thanksgiving. It was a joyous time, but there were always those twinges of sadness and loss. I was thankful for what had been saved, but what was lost was devastating.

My mother has recovered far beyond what the doctors ever predicted. She can walk without the aid of a cane, she drives a car, can take care of herself and has started to go back out into the world. It's hard for me to remember what she was like before her stroke. There are my childhood memories, but most of my adult life she has been handicapped. The adjustments have not been without considerable pain. The acceptance has been even more difficult. Kari, Eric and I live with the knowledge that we also may experience a stroke.

The family has survived; at times the challenge seemed impossible. If my parents hadn't stayed together, I don't think the family would have either. My father is very brave. After realizing a lot of things, I found that he is as courageous as my mother because he could have walked away from all the hurt and the sickness but didn't. My mother is a testimony, and watching her walk around the house says it all after knowing where she had started from five years ago. But there will always be the resentment and the anger at what fate has dealt us. I think that that is just a part of being alive and having survived a trauma like this. There are still a lot of things I have to deal with, but time has healed wounds and given me an insight that few people my age have. It has made me stronger, realizing that I have strengths inside me that I never thought I could ever have had.

from the Stroke Connection January/February 1988

A Locker Room Pep Talk

by "Black Jack" Tinson, Upland, California

Senility is a term so often used to break down old people—to get them to fade into the clouds of despair before they leave this mortal vale of remorse! Do not give up! FIGHT as though you were 20 again. I.Q. is nothing but what your brain recalled at a particular time! I think slowing down mentally with the advancing years is all a myth; it can place you in a lethargic state—if you permit it!

Here are some things you can do to keep yourself active:

1. First of all, WRITE—just anything; your family history or your autobiography. Write down your thoughts or write about your friends.

2. Play cards—bridge, poker, gin or any type of game. Make up a group to come in for an afternoon or an evening. (Peggy, my darling angel—my wife, arranges this for me.)

3. Organize your mind; jot down things of interest to you.

4. Keep a daily diary—it doesn't have to be long—of special events that took place in the world, or what happened to you today!

5. Repeat all instructions—say them aloud to yourself. This will help you remember much better.

6. I really believe this: Put away the calculator. Do your figuring by hand; add, subtract, multiply on paper or, best of all, in your head.

7. Break up things into similar categories. On your grocery list, for example, group things as canned goods, meat or paper goods.

8. Do things in sequence, organize yourself, think through every task. Save steps, manpower and your head!

9. Read as much as you can. Learn to read fast—this will keep your mind sharp and involve practically all of your brain!

10. Develop your critical thinking! I did this in my class room and on the practice field of football. Here is an example: If I asked you to go to the creek with a 5-gallon and a 7 gallon jar, and bring me exactly three gallons back with guess work, how would you do it? Use all of the water you wish! Analyzing the procedure improves one's mind!

11. Try to learn to play the organ or piano.

12. Watch and describe a sunset and what it means to you.

13. Make a list of your good qualities.

14. Try to laugh each day—especially at yourself.

15. Express appreciation to your loved ones.

16. Meditate a little each day.

17. Listen to the rain or wind.

18. Eat out at a nice restaurant. Eat by candlelight (Peg insists that we do). It works wonders.

19. Read a good novel.

20. Take frequent naps.

21. Have friends take you to a zoo. Take a boat ride on a river or the ocean.

22. Daydream—but not too much; you must not be unrealistic.

23. Try to write some poetry.

24. Sit by a fireplace that is glowing.

25. Visit someone in the hospital (but don't stay too long!)

26. Find something good in everyone you meet.

27. Have fun! BE CHEERFUL!

28. Live a little—thank God you are here each morning.

29. Be good to yourself—you deserve it.
30. Relax a little each day.
31. Do not sit for long intervals—get up often and move around if possible.
32. Eat slowly and not too much.
33. Have a happy hour of vegetables, cheese and crackers; perhaps, one cocktail.
34. Also, eat plenty of fruit and whole grain cereals.
35. Do not attempt to repair dentures or bridges; use a professional dentist.
36. Remember most headaches are caused by tension; try to release them by deep breathing.
37. Decide what is fun for you, then do it!
38. Rest often, be moderate in all things; we can overdo those things in which we become interested; there is tomorrow—don't forget! Plan for it.

All of these could apply to stroke survivors, too. I have tried to follow most of these rules after I lost my right leg, had three heart attacks, two strokes and numerous surgical procedures. A loving family around me and close friends gave me courage and inspired me to succeed!

The above article is very simple, but we must remember that strokes will often last a lifetime. Those of us who are survivors must prevent boredom, depression and loneliness! YOU ARE ALIVE, AREN'T YOU? BUCK-UP AND FIGHT—make the best of a bad situation! It is tough, but follow the easy rules above and begin to live again! FIGHT ON! FIGHT ON!

Editor's note: Have you figured out the answer to number 10? Fill the five gallon jar and pour it into the seven gallon jar. Fill the five gallon jar again and pour it into the seven gallon—only two gallons will fit into the jar leaving three gallons in the five gallon jar.

from the Stroke Connection September/October 1987

A Mandate for Change

by Gennie Barnett, Seattle, Washington

When I left the hospital, someone advised me, "Now, you want to do everything you can to reorganize your life just the way it was before your stroke." Not only was that impossible to do, but it would have been a mistake to attempt it. The key to coping with a major crisis in one's life is to view it as a mandate for change. One door has closed. Instead of pounding on the closed door, why not look for another opening?

Major crises afford us a wonderful opportunity to ponder the direction of our life, examine our goals and make corrections in our course. It is folly to attempt to return to our former situation or to try to recreate the past. Although we may not recognize it, we have changed irrevocably, as have the circumstances about us. There is something new and exciting awaiting us, if only we have the eyes to see it. This requires letting go of the old life, the old way of doing things. St. Paul refers to "the removing of those things that are shaken, that those things which cannot be shaken may remain," (Hebrews 12:24). Significantly, the god Shiva is the god of both destruction and creation. The destruction that comes into our lives is often a form of housecleaning preliminary to moving in some new and richer furnishings.

This is not easy. It involves time and tears and endless patience. Fortunately, most of us are handed a large hunk of time as a free gift for our recuperation. We must discover that grace which will enable us to accept the present situation and forget the past. Every card player knows that the cardinal rule of the game is that you must play the hand you have been dealt. If we complain about the cards we have been dealt, we will find ourselves out of the game, alone and embittered.

I am sure that many people pity me because I am so obviously severely disabled as a result of my stroke. Despite the fact that my wings have been clipped, I feel that this is the happiest and most productive period of my life in many ways. In the seven years since my stroke, I have taken two correspondence courses over a period of four years. For the past five years I have done volunteer work out of my home in excess of 40 hours a week, which has bolstered my self-esteem.

But the real change has been inside. I see the world in a different way and have new values. I have learned much and made so many new discoveries. Best of all, I have rid myself of fear and can face the future with confidence. Each day I learn something new, something more I can contribute. Scarcely a week passes without a minor epiphany that enlarges my understanding of the world. My disability has not dispossessed me. Life is good.

from the Stroke Connection May/June 1988

A Speech Pathologist's Story

by Elaine Argetsinger, St. Louis Park, Minnesota
with assistance from Cindy Busch, Shorewood, Minnesota

Twenty years ago I was a speech pathologist in the Hopkins public schools in Minnesota. After a school meeting on February 1, 1968, I got into my car and started for home. I got up to the highway and I suddenly felt funny. I parked the car and heard, "Are you all right, Elaine?" It was the teacher from the car behind me. I blacked out and stayed in a coma for 10 days. When I came to, I found that I couldn't speak. I tried to move and found out that my right side was paralyzed down to my toes. I just lay there —I couldn't write or read, although I could understand what people said. For seven weeks I was in the hospital. I had speech therapy but it wasn't like it is today. I do remember the Language Master. For days I would say after the model, "leg, leg, leg—arm, arm, arm—body, body, body." It is the one thing I can remember.

At home, the laborious task of learning to do things again began. After seven weeks my right leg was stronger, so I was mobile to some extent. I had a two-story house with all bedrooms and the bathroom on the second floor. I made it but it was hard. We needed extra help around the house for two months.

Within three months when I was stronger, I tackled the sewing machine. I used to make all my own clothes. Now I couldn't remember anything, not even how the sewing machine worked. I couldn't read, so the patterns meant nothing. So I started with a skirt I had made, took it apart and put it back together again. It was hard work. Today I make all of my own clothes again.

Within the year, I joined the Women's Alliance of my church, which met twice a month. There were many friends who took me to those meetings. I worked on many crafts and became more and more skilled at them. We also had a play reading group. I can remember my silence when the others took their turns. It was many years before I was able to read the plays. I just listened. Recently, I was a program chairman for the Alliance monthly meetings. I still go to these meetings and I do participate.

And then there were the speech pathologists—they were a great help, both with speech and providing support. When I got home from the hospital, I had speech lessons once a week from a speech pathologist who came to the house. I also had speech help from a retired pathologist who was a good friend. When summer came, I went to the University Hospital for more speech sessions. The 1969 fall meeting of the Minnesota Speech and Hearing Association was all about strokes. I was interviewed on stage about my experiences after having a stroke and becoming aphasic. Even though it had been 20 months since my stroke and I still couldn't speak well, the audience seemed to find my personal story very interesting and ironic.

That fall I found I couldn't read more than a first-grade book. When I was taking my degree in speech pathology, I also took many reading courses, and later worked at Macalaster College in St. Paul, Minnesota, as a speed reading teacher. So I knew I had a serious problem. I went to the public library, took out a number of books—easy books, first-grade books—and I started. I borrowed the Reading Laboratory from our school in Hopkins, and the rest was plain hard work. For two years I struggled with it. Today I can read adult novels.

Then there was the piano. I had practiced for years, and had at one time dreamed of being a concert pianist. I had thought that I would play to my heart's content when I retired. The stroke changed all that. The left hand was all right, but the right hand wouldn't work properly. I realized I needed new interests and activities. I searched around until I found a painting class with the Senior Program of St. Louis Park, Minnesota. I took up oil and water color painting. It filled a gap and I became more and more adept at it. I've had about seven or eight exhibits. For the past four years, I have been an art coordinator for the Metropolitan Senior Federation of Minnesota. I also worked on weaving woolen rugs for our living and dining rooms. I wove two large ones and a lot of little ones. They are beautiful and a joy to behold. They are the results of the crafts I learned to do at church.

My favorite pastime has been traveling. I have traveled with my husband, my daughter and son-in-law, my son and with friends. I have been to Alaska, England, Scotland, France, Switzerland, Italy, Germany, Scandinavia, Russia, Hong Kong and the Island of McCau.

In the last year or two, I have taken a course at Courage Center on peer counseling. I became a peer counselor for stroke survivors and their families. I go to Methodist Hospital in St. Louis Park, Minnesota once a week and I counsel about six or eight stroke families each time. Our primary responsibility is to listen to the stroke survivors and to give them strength to cope with the changes in their lives. I really enjoy helping these people.

About four years ago, I started to make frequent speaking appearances in front of stroke support groups. I told about my experiences as a speech pathologist who had become aphasic. My husband and I also were interviewed by a cable TV program and we participated in a local TV talk show on behalf of the Courage Stroke Network. People always seem interested that even a speech pathologist can have a stroke and become aphasic. I do feel that my background as a speech pathologist has helped in my struggle to regain my speech.

from the Stroke Connection September/October 1987

A Tribute to Our "Unsung Heroes"

by Vivian Larson, Sheboygan, Wisconsin

They never made the big headlines, nor are they ever presented with a large gold trophy, but in the stroke world they rank right up there with the doctors, nurses, and therapists. I am speaking of those who uncomplainingly take on the role of caregiver for a stroke survivor. It may be a spouse, some other family member, or just a very good friend. Whoever it is, he deserves more praise than we, as stroke survivors, will ever be able to express.

First of all, let me say how difficult it must have been for my husband, the caregiver, to see me, a once very active and healthy loved one, suffering from the effects, great or small, of a stroke. Children and grandchildren too realized the problem, but everyone involved gradually accepted the inevitable and went about helping me get on with my life. A stroke may result in role reversal for a husband and wife, as in my case, wherein my husband not only does what he is accustomed to doing, but also does what I am unable to do now. He has to draw on an extra supply of patience and courage to do this satisfactorily for both of us. Of course, I must use a lot of patience with him as well when he doesn't do things the way I would have done them. Remember, he's doing his best at jobs he's never been responsible for before. My husband gives constant encouragement to me. He doesn't do things for me that we both know I can do for myself. Then, too, he will sometimes leave little things undone hoping that I will accept the challenge and try to do them myself. If I can't, then he will do them.

My husband tends to his own health by having regular checkups by his doctor. In this way he keeps fit for the caregiving job which has become his lot in life.

He may be called upon to do the laundry and says thanks to modern science for fabrics which require little or no ironing. Shopping for groceries and other items is also included in his routine, especially if I have trouble walking. He hires help if it's available with housecleaning and also the yard work — lawn mowing and snow removal.

He and I plan together for Christmas and birthday gifts for children and grandchildren. We do a lot of catalog shopping which makes it easier for both of us.

He encourages me to get out and go places even though I might not want to go. He plans outings in which both of us can participate.

He keeps up with his own life outside the home. He remains active in clubs and attends various invitational functions, but is always sure that I know what to do in case of an emergency. He knows that it is good for his own mental health to withdraw from the role of a caregiver occasionally for an evening or afternoon or once in a while even for a weekend.

We continue in hobbies which we enjoyed together before the CVA which brought changes to our lives.

Much of what I have written is affected by my own personal experience as a stroke survivor with a very caring husband. However, some of it will apply to others in similar circumstances. Each stroke is different and thus it determines the direction which our future life takes.

So let's all honor our caregivers with a standing ovation. Those who can't stand may just sit and give a sharp salute (your choice of right or left hand) to these brave people. They are truly the "unsung heroes" of the stroke world and without them, we stroke survivors would be lost.

from Stroke Connection July/August 1985

A Young Woman's Struggle with Stroke

by Judy Hopia, Maple Plain, Minnesota

One cold November night in 1972, the unbelievable happened to me, a healthy, 24-year-old, athletic and physically fit mother of two. I had a stroke. People say "This sort of thing happens to old people; it does not happen to a young mother."

Life was grand for us before it happened. My husband had just been promoted, we had a 4-year-old girl, Kris, and a six-month-old baby boy, Jay. We had just bought our first home, and the American dream was well within reach.

To help make ends meet, I worked 30 to 40 hours a week as a beautician. On days I didn't work, I took care of another child for pay and for companionship for my 4-year-old. In spite of being extremely busy, I kept my home immaculate. People were amazed by my energy level, and I burst with pride.

But on a Sunday in November, I was stripped of all use of the left half of my body. I felt it was perhaps God's way of harshly telling me that there is no such thing as a "superwoman."

I survived, but was severely limited by the paralysis on my left side. Friends and family made it a point to stop by and help and marvel at how well I was coming along. They were amazed at how well Kris, only 4, could help me enough so that I didn't have to hire someone to help with housework. But it hurt my pride to see that my 4-year-old and my nine-month-old were more physically capable than I was.

My recovery was remarkable the first year. I progressed from the doctors saying, "I don't think she will live," to "I can't promise she'll ever be out of a wheelchair," to "it would be a miracle if she can ever walk unaided." But in September 1973, I walked into my daughter's kindergarten class without my cane. The praise I got from my friends, family and doctors inspired me. But the hope of total recovery was my driving force.

Soon after I accomplished that feat, a tremor developed in my left arm. The tremor had a "one-two" polka beat that was very accurate, 24 hours a day. It was exhausting and came on top of a pain in my arm caused by thalamic nerve damage. After tranquilizers and psychiatric help failed, I agreed to some risky brain surgery which was fairly successful and allowed me to get on with my life.

The years passed, and I promised myself and my friends that my recovery would go on, but it was all talk. I entered college. I was only an average student before, but during my first quarter I earned a 3.5 grade point average, in the second quarter a 4.0! But "superwoman" crashed again, and I spent six weeks in a mental rehabilitation ward.

There I met a nurse who taught me that improving my self-esteem was impossible as long as I loved only the right (good) half of me. My stroke had made me psychologically detached from the left side of my body, and I often referred to my useless left arm as "this thing."

She told me to think of the sides of my body as twin children; one good twin and one bad twin, and how I had to accept and love the "bad" half of my body. I could finally grasp my left arm and weep for the hatred, abuse and rejection I had felt for it.

I spent hours in self-esteem therapy with physically able-bodied people, who couldn't understand my physical and emotional deficits, fears and frustrations. I expressed my frustration to my nurse and she told me about the Courage Stroke Network, a support group for people who have had strokes and their families.

I attended my first meeting at Courage Center in Golden Valley. The other stroke people were a wonderful group of older adults with whom I tried to share my frustrations of being a stroke-involved wife and mother. But, like loving grandparents, they assured me how lucky my children and husband were that I had all my life and love ahead to give.

I met another young woman who had had a stroke, and we realized we needed a group our own age to share our special needs. With help from the Courage Stroke Network coordinator, we formed a group of people under the age of 50 to meet in my friend Jane's home in Minneapolis.

The encouragement and support we drew from each other was a source of strength that we were all so grateful to find. We shared concerns like "Do you ever have tears flow for no reason, sometimes inappropriately?" "Do you laugh at times when it is really appropriate to cry?" Do you recognize a friend's face one minute and the next minute try to figure out where you've seen the person before?" We can share these things with each other and laugh, while these occurrences wouldn't seem so funny to our healthy loved ones.

To psychologically recover from my stroke, I had to grieve, and cope with and learn from my grieving.

I have grieved for the fact that I put so much responsibility on my young children, demanding that they do tasks according to my instructions and burdening them with my disappointments when they didn't accomplish the tasks as well as I once did.

I grieved for the fact that I didn't have the ability to be an efficient mother to my baby boy, trying so often to pick him up in my arms only to squeeze him to tears or drop him back into the crib.

I grieved for the anxiety I felt toward my husband, knowing that somewhere out there, there were other women who could better meet the expectations and dreams he once had for me.

We stroke survivors shared these experiences with each other in the Courage Stroke Network, and after a time we felt the need to search out and share our experiences and support with people who recently had strokes, helping them within days or weeks of their strokes, rather than waiting for them to just "happen upon" our group.

In 1981, we formed a task force consisting of the Courage Stroke Network coordinator and representatives from several member stroke clubs and area institutions. We eventually created the Courage Stroke Network Peer Counselor Training Program. Stroke survivors and spouses go through an extensive training program so that they can visit and provide support to recently stroke involved people and their families. Each peer counselor is sponsored and supervised by an area hospital or other health care facility. Several metro area hospitals participate in the program, and it has received a warm response from stroke patients, hospital staff and volunteers.

It's been rewarding for me to work as a volunteer for the peer counselor program, to realize the goal of reaching stroke people soon after their strokes when they need our help the most. We let them know we are out there with them, struggling with some of the same feelings and frustrations, but struggling with as much courage as we can.

It's rewarding to let other stroke people know that climbing the mountain is worth all the "blood, sweat and tears." We tell them that they are needed. We encourage their efforts and understand their fears. I've been able to show myself, by showing them, that the struggle is worth it and there is life after a stroke.

from the Stroke Connection December 1980

After Your Stroke

by Art Greenough

"Dear Lord, please grant me the serenity to accept that which I cannot change, to change that which I can change, and the wisdom to know the difference."

Nearly everyone has heard this prayer. Alcoholics Anonymous has used it for years. Strokers would do well to take a page from A.A. and use this prayer. It says, loud and clear, "One day at a time...take things one day at a time."

After the first hours, days or weeks, you are once again able to figure out which end is up, but you are not ready yet to accept this new position in life.

What was done with ease before is hard now; hard, or in some cases, impossible. What to do? Take things one day at a time. Learn the framework in which you can live, in which you can work. Don't cuss God out because of this; just do as good as you can.

Let's face it—you're different. Your stroke has changed the way your body works. The brain damage has changed the way you think; possibly your whole outlook on life.

You may have had to switch roles with your spouse, or perhaps had to take on some of your spouse's traditional jobs in the family.

The important thing to remember is that your spouse will be taking things one day at a time also. Both your lives can then be that much easier. Things are not necessarily going to work out. Be prepared to try and accept.

"One day at a time." Try it. If you succeed, you will live again. The chances are that you will not be the person that you were, but you will be able to enjoy your life. You may not be sound of body, but you will be full of life.

from the Stroke Connection January 1984

Urban and Alice: Living with Stroke

by Alice Beer, St. Paul, Minnesota

The popular song that fall was, "Love is Lovelier the Second Time Around." It was their song. They were each marrying for the second time. He had lost his spouse to cancer. She had been widowed in World War II. They had met through their adult children and lived only two blocks apart. Anyway, it was a fortunate meeting. They were lucky, they felt. She had read somewhere that only one in 100 marry after age 45. They were both 45. So, without pomp and fanfare, they began their partnership. They were married at Thanksgiving time and they were truly thankful!

He had purchased a hardware store earlier that year—another dream realized. He loved working with his hands, helping others repair things really made his work rewarding. She helped him by running errands, doing the banking and the bookwork and sending out statements.

For nine years after their marriage things went well. They spoke often of how very fortunate they were. They worked and saved for retirement and for "a rainy day."

Then one evening in early fall, without warning, he slumped over while watching television. She was in the kitchen only a few steps from the den. She found him on the floor making strange sounds. Hospitalization followed.

After many tests were done, he was diagnosed as having had a slight stroke. He recovered completely this time. After two weeks of rest he was back on the job with some part-time help, but what a scare they'd had!

It was so frightening to him that he decided that perhaps working so many hours wasn't very wise. Within two years he sold the hardware store. He stayed on for some time after the sale, however, to orient the new owner and to introduce him to the credit customers.

Following the sale, retirement was just great! "Like Christmas every day," he once said to her. She agreed! Finally, there was time to sit in the backyard under the apple tree. They would have their lunch there. Each fall he would go duck hunting, his favorite sport. She would occasionally play bridge and also kept busy sewing for the grandchildren.

About two years passed. One day, upon returning from their lake home, they discovered that their property had been vandalized for the third time in a short while. It was very upsetting for both of them, but especially so for him. While he was calling the police, she noticed that he was not able to find words to express what had happened. He was stammering and misusing words.

When the police arrived, they also noticed that he was not well.

Again, hospitalization followed. The doctor said that he was having symptoms of a stroke, although his vital signs were within normal limits and that they planned to observe him for a day or so. A day later, while in intensive care, a stroke did occur, resulting in aphasia and paralysis of his right side.

The next three weeks in the hospital and 18 months at home were filled with extensive therapy. He walked again and was able to use his good arm to paint the trim on their house. What an accomplishment!

The return of his speech was a bit more stubborn, although they were able to communicate quite effectively. He hesitated to go out socially because it was difficult for him to respond to questions.

Life changed in many other ways as well. He would never drive again; he would never pay the bills or write a check; he could not read, tell time or dial the telephone to call for help. She had become the caregiver. Her role had markedly changed.

At about that time, a representative from St. Mary's Rehabilitation Center contacted her about a possible support group for families of stroke-involved people. Involvement with that group helped her deal with her new role as caregiver, as well as dealing with problems such as possible over-protection, leaving him unattended and finding time for herself.

As time progressed she found she was able to leave him alone for short periods of time. Life had its frustrations but they learned to cope.

Five years later, he once again had a stroke. This time he had a clot in the spine—a really devastating stroke which left him paralyzed from the hips down. They were crushed and the tears came readily.

It became apparent that this 6'3" man could not be cared for at home. The realization that they would be forced to live apart was an intolerable blow. How could they resign themselves to this fact?

from the Stroke Connection February 1984

Urban and Alice

by Alice Beer, St. Paul, Minnesota

They often prayed together and some of their prayers were answered. He wouldn't be able to go home but he was accepted at Harmony Nursing Home, a skilled-care facility and her first choice after having seen many.

Harmony has staff and equipment as found in a hospital, yet has a warm and cheery home-like atmosphere. Even so, it was a big adjustment!

That adjustment has included many positive things. There's a new warmth in their relationship. They've found that here there is time for holding hands, for reminiscing over coffee, and for laughing a little.

She was especially pleased one day when on a visit she had to search for him. He was not on the second floor, in his room or in the lounge. To her utter amazement, she learned that he had propelled himself onto the elevator, down to the lobby and through double doors out to the patio. He'd had the incentive to do this on his own! He spent many summer hours on that patio, acquiring a tan and enjoying the outdoors, and eventually began doing some socializing. He was adjusting—a triumph for both of them!

They began joining other residents to say the rosary on Fridays with a group of dedicated ladies from St. Patrick's who would lead them.

They then started to participate in some planned activities and have found some contentment once again. He was stimulated by the activity and by all the especially pleasant and helpful staff. He started to say new words. One week she counted six new words. It seemed almost a miracle!

It wasn't long before indoor picnics with the family were planned at their home on Sundays with Metro Mobility being his mode of transportation. On alternating Sundays they would invite family or friends to dine at the nursing home with them in the little private dining room.

There have been ups and downs, but they knew these would occur and have learned to accept them. Just recently, a bout with infection sent him to the hospital again for a six-day stay. It was a setback— somewhat trying and discouraging, which left him in a weakened condition, but they are coping with this just as with earlier setbacks.

Their goal now is to someday live again under the same roof in their stucco home with the red trim he painted. Home, where he might live more independently. Home, where they might share the togetherness they so cautiously planned over 18 years ago.

Eighteen years ago when the lyrics of OUR song were:

"Who can say what led us to this miracle we found—We're so glad we met the second time around."

I am Alice, Urban is my husband, and this is our story.

from the Stroke Connection June 1984

Alice and Urban at Home

by Alice Beer, St. Paul, Minnesota

The buds on their beloved apple tree are a deep pink now and soon the fragrance of their blossoms will fill the air. Sitting there, underneath, at the white picnic table is Urban in his "four-wheeler." He is enjoying lunch with his spouse. A picnic for two, so much like it was years ago, soon after retirement and years before his stroke. Similar in a way, and yet so different. They are more aware of the peace and beauty surrounding them—the green grass, the beautiful blue sky, the birds and the hum of a bumble bee.

Urban's realm is their six-room house, the yard, the recently installed ramp and the screened-in back porch. Somehow this seems to suffice. It is an independence and a freedom they prayed for so often during the 12 months he was in the nursing home.

Urban was transferred from the hospital to the nursing home in April 1983, and as early as October, Alice became actively involved in finding help to get him home. A good friend suggested that she attend a seminar on home issues and services, two of which she subsequently used: Supportive Care to the Elderly and Alternative Care Program.

After hearing about the latter program, she contacted them and was told she and Urban would not qualify because their savings were above the limit allowed. It was very frustrating. They had always been frugal and now were guilty of having a small savings account! The irony of it was that their funds were rapidly dwindling because of the huge costs at the nursing home. Understandably, she felt dejected and had sleepless nights. Also, she felt they were discriminated against for saving their money for "that rainy day." So sad, so disappointing. Somehow, she could not allow things to rest that way.

In February, she knew that she had to find her own help and pay for it. he prepared a list of possible health aids, therapists, etc., along with the days and times she would need them. Urban's doctor then gave his consent for Urban to return home.

Busy days followed. Alice rented the needed equipment—a hospital bed with rails, a wheelchair, a Hoyer lift, an air pump and an alternating pressure mattress. Their goals were beginning to be realized. Urban came home April 1, 1984, as scheduled.

All necessary care and services are provided by an occupational therapist, a public health nurse, a licensed practical nurse and home health aide who come to the house on a scheduled basis. Besides her regular household responsibilities, Alice coordinates and supervises this busy schedule and, being a registered nurse herself, completes many of the medical responsibilities.

At home now, some days still hold frustrations and difficulties. Somehow, sharing them does lighten their impact. Discouraging talk is banned. Well, almost. At any rate they do make an effort to not dwell on the "negatives."

A message to those of you reading this story who are, perhaps, in a similar situation because of a stroke: Being hopeful and never "giving up" has helped so much to cope. We did get much needed help because we searched for it. It is there to be had, but you have to "go after it." We are Urban and Alice living at home now with stroke. God love you.

from the Stroke Connection April 1988

Alive and Kicking!

by John Mastel, Vadnais Heights, Minnesota

"*You are so lucky to be alive. I had an uncle who had an aneurysm and he died...*"

"*...My dad had one of those and he lived for about two weeks after they did brain surgery on him. We don't think he ever knew what happened to him..*"

"*...Tom did the strangest things after his operation for the aneurysm. He was just never the same again, poor guy.*"

I swear that some people think with their feet, not with their brains. These are a few of the comments made to me by well-intentioned people after I suffered a rupture of an aneurysm and subsequent stroke seven years ago. Even while I was lying in a hospital bed not knowing what had happened to me, people were telling me how lucky I was in comparison to other people they had known. Suddenly, it seemed everyone knew of somebody who had had an aneurysm, ruptured or otherwise, and had not survived to tell about it. All these "victims" were spoken of in the past tense; they had died. Not me. I am alive and kicking.

My problems started one mild January morning in 1981. The temperature was 32 degrees Fahrenheit and the sun was shining brightly. I had dropped a crew of men off at a job site, gotten them working on a project and left to satisfy a complaint from a homeowner on a house completed about six weeks before. Being the owner of a construction company, I wanted my customers to be as happy as possible with the contracted work. The complaint was an easy one to remedy. It required a small section of flashing and drip cap be resecured above a third-story window on the front of the house. I arrived, placed a sturdy aluminum ladder against the house, put on a tool belt and climbed up the ladder to start the repair. While I was securing the drip cap, the legs of the ladder let go without warning. They slid out from under me and caused me, my tools and the ladder

28

to come crashing down. I remember the fall very vividly, having my whole life flash before me. The fall seemed to take an eternity, everything happening in super slow motion. I remember thinking, please God, don't let this hurt too much. If I'm going to die, please make it fast. Don't let me suffer too long. Falling down headfirst, tools flying all over, I remember thinking about my wife, my children, my parents, my dogs. My hands instinctively went out in front of me to attempt to break the fall. With a loud thud, I landed headfirst, arms extended, on a concrete sidewalk. I lay on the sidewalk in a heap, a ball of human mass, with no movement. Probably more unconscious than conscious, I remember thinking if this is what being dead is, it is not so bad. I felt no pain. My whole body was numb. I could not move and my vision was blurred. I remember after some time passed (I have no idea how much) a woman standing over me just looking. If she spoke, I did not know it. She just looked. Suddenly, I heard the yelp of a siren. It was the paramedics.

Four firemen got out of the shining red van and walked toward me. I heard one of them ask the woman if she knew what had happened here. She said, "I was standing on my front porch across the street waiting for my dog, Nellie, to finish her "duty" when I heard this loud crashing sound, like metal hitting concrete. I also heard a man yell some obscenities which I just cannot repeat. You know the kind I mean! Anyway, I looked over here and saw this man falling to the ground from up there, that third-story window. That's when I called you people 'cause you are the best. You can help him, can't you? I think he is still alive.'"

With that the fireman left the woman and walked over to me. He stood by the other firemen and said, "The lady says he fell from up by the third-story window. Falling that far, he may have a broken neck or back. Jim, you get the backboard. We'll strap him on the backboard and transport that way to Ramsey. Anybody know who the poor bastard is?" No one answered. With that they put me on a backboard and loaded me into the van.

I tried to talk, but it was as if no one could hear me or understand me. En route to the hospital, the firemen were busy trying to keep me secure on the backboard. They had four straps holding me down.

They put a big air bag, clear plastic, around my left arm. I heard one of the firemen say, "I'll inflate an air splint on the left arm; that will keep it immobile till the doctors decide what to do with it. Must be busted in at least five or six places. I think the shoulder is broken too. If his back is broken, he'll probably be paralyzed." The other firemen agreed.

We arrived at St. Paul Ramsey Hospital where I was wheeled into the emergency room. After being poked, prodded, pulled and pricked by countless cold silvery instruments, the doctors said they needed to examine me more thoroughly. They had to remove me from the backboard. Very carefully they started to unstrap me and then lift me onto a hospital gurney. As soon as I was secure on the gurney, I was taken into a room for x-rays. The technician must have taken 25 or 30 x-rays — she had a picture of every last part of my skeleton. After the x-rays, I must have passed out. The next thing I knew, it was a Tuesday. My fall had occurred on a Thursday. What I did not know was that almost four weeks had passed in between that Thursday and this Tuesday

What happened was—besides having broken my left arm in five places, shattering my left shoulder, breaking three ribs, and having multiple lacerations—I had ruptured an aneurysm in my brain. The doctors, having determined that I was hemorrhaging in my brain, rushed me into surgery first for an emergency angiogram with contrast, then stabilized me and proceeded to perform brain surgery. They had to shave my head, cut my skull open from the middle of the forehead to the top of the head to below the left ear. They located the aneurysm and placed two metal clips of one and one-half inches each on the aneurysm, successfully halting the hemorrhage. Completing the procedure, the doctors closed my skull by using large one inch metal staples for the length of the incision. The staples looked like the ties of a railroad track as they were inserted around my head. A very strange sight indeed.

Having survived the fall, then the ruptured aneurysm and surgery to repair it, I was informed by the doctors I had also had a stroke. Somehow a cerebral vascular accident had occurred. Something had gone wrong with the circulation of blood to the brain cells and my brain had been injured. The damages to the brain, or "deficits" as they are called, were significant. They are too numerous to list here; suffice it to say my life has been changed in some very dramatic ways.

No longer do I own and operate a business, working 80 plus hours a week. The business had to be sold along with the equipment. My priorities changed. Now I serve on the staff of a local hospital as a stroke counselor, hopefully giving to other stroke survivors the encouragement and example they can use to overcome their "deficits." Hard work and determination can make a difference in one's rehabilitation. Life can be meaningful after stroke.

from the Stroke Connection September 1985

An Outbound Experience

by Jeanette Weeks, Minneapolis, Minnesota

I have been involved in stroke clubs for several years now and I can laugh at my first experience with a stroke club. However, at the time I was not laughing. I was close to tears because I was frightened about going out in public.

My peer counselor had arranged for a member of the Survivors' Stroke Club to pick me up to attend a holiday party. I was reluctant to get involved because I was so self-conscious about how I looked. I told my peer counselor that I would rather not attend the meeting and venture out in public yet. She and my therapists tried to convince me to go out, but I was stubborn.

I did not write down the date or time of the event and so when Jane arrived to pick me up to attend the outing, I was taken by surprise; so much in fact that I didn't have any concrete reason as to why I couldn't go. So I left with Jane to go to the party. I was very scared and nervous. At that time, I was using a quad cane and my balance was poor. Jane tried to get me to relax by talking about her own stroke experience. I asked many questions.

When we arrived at the restaurant, there was a steep curb in front of the entrance. I tried to lift my weak leg high enough to step over it, but I fell down and my cane went flying through the air. I did not have the strength to lift myself up. All I could do was laugh hysterically, but I wanted to cry. Jane told me I had to try to help as she was not strong enough to get me up. Meanwhile, a crowd started to gather around me. I was very embarrassed.

Much to my surprise, my adrenalin was pumping so much that I got myself up to an erect position. I wobbled into the lobby section of the restaurant, sat down to recover and noticed that my pant leg was ripped and my paralyzed leg had a big cut at the knee. Naturally, it did not hurt because I had no feeling in that leg.

Jane walked with me into the dining room and graciously introduced me to everyone. When I first glanced at the room which had been sectioned off, I thought it might be a meeting of Jaycees or Kiwanis, because everyone looked so normal to me. My feelings of self-consciousness soon dissipated as I started to talk to people. My peer counselor was thrilled that I came. When I told her of my grand entrance into the building, she remarked, "Well, you did it." As I talked to more people, I began to relax. Never before had I felt more accepted and welcomed by a group of strangers.

When the waiter brought the bill, one of the leaders of the group noticed an error. He asked, "Who in this room can do math?" It turned out the spouses of the stroke survivors figured out the bill and, indeed, there was a mistake by the waiter. We all enjoyed the evening. Everyone was especially kind to me and said how brave I was to attend a stroke club function so soon after my stroke. Later that night, when I was back in my safe and secure environment, I remembered laughing with other stroke survivors. I discovered that while it is safe to be back, it is not as much fun.

The next day I could hardly wait to tell my physical therapist and my sister about my accomplishments. I could not wait until the next meeting of the stroke club.

Since that time, I have regained my strength and I go to as many stroke club events as possible. The camaraderie of the stroke survivors is so enjoyable and comforting.

I wanted to tell you about my experience so that you will know that, yes, it is scary to branch out of your safe, secure environment. But if you don't make an effort, you will be missing out on new challenges. Almost everyone feels scared and nervous at their first stroke club meeting. But I guarantee you that you will feel welcomed and not alone if you at least go.

from the Stroke Connection March 1982

Arm

by Kristen Naylor

I know I am paralyzed

in my right arm.

It doesn't bother

me much . . . .

but . . . .

I dream of two arms.

I realize

that I have to face the fact . . . .

the fact

that it's not going to be

easy at all.

from the Stroke Connection March 1982

Frustration

by Kristen Naylor

What a hassle

it is

to get out . . . .

a simple letter.

from the Stroke Connection November 1988

Caregiving during the Holidays
A Caregiver's Perspective

by Alice Beer, St. Paul, Minnesota

Another holiday season is fast approaching. Ten year's ago, after my husband's stroke, we wondered how we could ever be happy without the hurry and scurry and preparation for the family at our table Christmas Day.

How could we possibly be content without the large Christmas tree? How different not to have him place the star on the tree, without a step stool to reach the top. He would miss checking all the little lights before distributing them evenly on all the branches. All this to be done before the very old, antique and fragile ornaments would be hung—ornaments that we both had fallen heir to from our individual families over the years—so precious, so unique!

We did survive that change. There have been other changes that have been more difficult to accept. We know, after all, that there would always be a Christmas, even though it was changed for us in many ways.

Perhaps, now, the full meaning of the joyous season has become more defined. We aren't able to hurry and scurry about and, somehow, it isn't expected of us now. We can now sit quietly and thoroughly enjoy this meaningful season...this season which is packed with nostalgia and never-ending joyful memories and song!

Happy Holidays!

from the Stroke Connection November 1988

Caregiving during the Holidays
A Professional's Perspective

by Jane Royse, Wilder Foundation, St. Paul, Minnesota

Yes, the holiday season is approaching and we're all probably asking ourselves if we'll survive yet another year. Survival may be even more of an issue if you're a family caregiver looking towards (notice I didn't say "forward to") the added stress and craziness the holidays can bring.

Some of you, like Alice, have redefined your expectations for the season and for yourself. You are clear as to what you can and cannot do and refuse to be caught in the "no-win" situation of scurrying about and still not getting everything done you wanted. For those of you who fit into this redefined behavioral category—give yourself a pat on the back and be applauded by the other category, "The Rest of the World", who still think that the holiday tradition of giving to others has to be at the expense of oneself. For that, "rest of the world", category, already overwhelmed just anticipating the added stress of the upcoming season, I'd like to suggest some ways to "fine-tune" your coping strategies so you'll do more than just survive the coming months.

1. Set realistic limits and stick to them! Caregivers have a tendency to answer all requests, no matter how unreasonable. During the holidays, feelings of anger or resentments are likely to occur when we feel others expect even more from us and we can't say no. While you might think your responsibility is to others, you are equally responsible to yourself.

2. Concentrate on what you *can* do, not what you *can't* do! Caregiving has probably brought about many changes in your life.

The holidays are reminders of how things used to be, but cannot be again. It's easy to drag ourselves down thinking about the past. Spend that time and energy making new memories that can be just as wonderful as the old ones.

3. When family or friends ask you what you want your present to be this year, tell them! Instead of saying the usual "I don't need anything" or "There's really nothing I want," give them suggestions of things you really could use. Someone to stay with Charlie while you have a weekend away, or someone who would take both of you for an occasional ride so you could sit back, enjoy the time and not always have to drive...two great gift ideas that would be easy to give, great to receive, but not often mentioned.

The holiday times can't be avoided! The only way we reach January is to go through November and December.I hope by using these suggestions you will enter 1989 with pleasant memories of the '88 holiday season and you will have developed some new coping techniques that will make your caregiving role and your life easier throughout the years to come.

from the Stroke Connection December 1981

Coping with Holiday Feasting and Fussing

by Marion Rasmussen, St. Paul, Minnesota

I was discharged from the hospital on November 7, 1973, so Thanksgiving was my first experience with a holiday after my stroke.

I cannot recall very much about the first Thanksgiving but what I do remember vividly was the bombardment of cross-conversation at the dinner table. Conversation on a one-to-one basis was difficult enough because of my aphasia, but trying to function in a room with more than two people was disastrous for me. Even though I was not speaking, the conversation of others at the table disturbed me and exhausted me so that I left soon after dinner. After 8 years, I still have problems conversing when there are other people within my hearing range. My only solution is to try to detach myself as much as possible from the group or try to fake my apparent participation by simply nodding and smiling.

Because I am clumsy and accident-prone, I have also, on occasion, asked my hostess to remove any precious china and stemware.

I learned some valuable things since that first Thanksgiving and coped with Christmas better. Christmas shopping was done from a wheelchair but in the middle of the week, rather than on a weekend and as soon as the store opened. I told several very kind clerks that I had aphasia and asked them to help me. Most of my shopping was done in several hours. The rest was done by family members or friends. I still do much of my shopping through catalogs and over the telephone, first explaining to the clerk that I have aphasia and have a communication problem. By explaining my problem, the clerks are much more willing to help me.

Gift-wrapping that first Christmas was a breeze. All gifts were boxed at the time of purchase so there was no need for gift wrapping. I am a pack-rat and had saved some gold elastic bands which I used instead of ribbon and bows. Gold elastic cord can be purchased in hobby shops or in the needle-art section of most department stores. Fashion a band by cutting a length of cord and tie a knot and slip the band over the package.

Sending Christmas cards was out of the question that first year. My very kind daughters sent short notes to my closest friends explaining the reason I was not able to send my own cards. Now I start writing cards early in November and have shortened the list considerably.

As far as entertaining is concerned, I find it very stressful and have tried to cope by planning ahead and falling back on tried-and-true recipes that can be prepared ahead of time, stored in the freezer and "prettied up" and made elegant at the time of serving. Most of my entertaining is for family members, and even though I am more relaxed, I still find it tiring. Fine china and stemware stay on the shelf while I use more serviceable tableware that goes into the dishwasher. Guests are free to help in the kitchen if they desire. I'll take any help I can get!

Cleaning house for the holidays or even a weekly cleaning is a problem for a handicapped person, unless one has the money to hire help. I have become more able since that first Christmas, but I can remember sitting on a chair dusting the chair and everything within reach, with one hand, then moving to another chair and repeating the process until the room was dusted as much as I was able. Also, closed doors shut out untidy rooms.

One note of humor. We have an artificial tree. That first Christmas I was trying so hard not to be on the sidelines—I wanted to participate as much as possible so I wanted to help trim the tree. With one hand on my cane and a bauble in my good hand, I attempted to place the ornament on a branch, and fell smack into the tree, breaking it. The tree was mended, of course, but I no longer trim the tree. We laugh now when we recall that Christmas, but tempers were short during that period and it was not funny then, but I have long since been forgiven, but the episode has not been forgotten.

from the Stroke Connection November/December 1984

Coping with Loneliness

by John Steenerson, Minneapolis, Minnesota

L oneliness can be a very ugly thing, and people like myself who have had a stroke, can experience this same feeling of ugliness. Or, perhaps, it is a feeling of alienation rather than loneliness. Whatever it is, it is a feeling which many people misinterpret.

Professionals, family members and friends sometimes interpret these feelings as feeling sorry for one's self or seeking sympathy or pity. However, in many cases this is not true.

I know from my own experience with stroke that people just did not understand what I was feeling. It was very difficult for me to stop and realize that the things I did before my stroke, I could no longer do.

At the same time, I think it was very hard for people close to me and the people working with me to realize that I just wanted everything to be the way it was before my stroke. And it was not. I began to feel very lonely, even though I was around people. I needed something more.

The answer lay right before me, but I was not able to see it. Eventually it came to me and I knew what I had to do. It was so easy and yet so difficult! I just had to be active! Activity was the answer I was looking for. It could be as simple as going for a ride in a car or sitting in the front yard watching the squirrels play or the wind blowing through the trees.

One day I got on a friend's bicycle—and God knows how scared I was. I rode a block and I could feel this big ol' smile come to my face. I was so happy to feel active again.

Then I went swimming and once again I felt fear. I stepped into the water and started walking deeper and deeper into the pool until the water was up to my neck. I don't know if I ever felt so afraid in my whole life. Then I actually started to swim. I could still do it, and it made me so happy to know that! Then I realized, beyond any doubt, I just needed to be active and the more active I became, the less lonely I felt. It has made me feel so good to know that once again the sky is the limit.

from the Stroke Connection August 1981

Faces of a Stroke

by Art Greenough

A stroke has many faces, depending upon one's vantage point. In my nearly six decades of life, I have seen five strokes, and each face was different, vastly different.

The first, when I was a youngster, did not leave too much of an impression. At fourteen, death is a foreign thing, neither understood nor, to a great degree, accepted. Death? To me or my family? Impossible!

The second encounter was at age 40. Death and dying were no longer foreign nor unbelievable. I had seen them too many times.

The next stroke, *I* was the one that was in the hospital. I was the one that the medical teams were fighting to save. This was a vastly different view point.

The next one was, to me, strictly hearsay, as I received the news long after it happened. It merely confirmed that death and stroke could— and often did—go hand in hand.

The last time, however, I was close enough to see the results. Worse, I was now well-enough acquainted with it to be able to read the possible result. It was a bleak picture.

Beverly's father suffered a massive cerebral hemorrhage, causing a stroke of right involvement. And I could see all kinds of nasty things in store for him.

While I didn't want to see him die, I was relieved at his death. After seventy-nine years, I doubt that he could have adjusted to life in a wheelchair. The right-sided stroke could have robbed him of speech as well.

The night before his death, Bev prayed. That prayer sums it up the best: "My dear Lord, please heal Dad. But Lord, if you can't heal him, then please take him home."

Amen.

from the Stroke Connection March 1982

Forever

by Kristen Naylor

I have

to be like this,

forever.

No holidays,

No pardon.

from the Stroke Connection December 1988

He Never
Walks Alone

by Linda McGerr, RPT, Courage Center,
Golden Valley, Minnesota

Hal Lance was honored with the Rose and Jay Phillips Award on October 4, 1988, four years after a stroke, a stroke that altered his plans but did not overcome his ambition. The Phillips Award, presented by Courage Center, recognizes individuals with disabilities who have achieved outstanding success in their vocations.

Carolyn Hardy, a job placement coordinator at Courage Center, had the opportunity to work with Hal and nominated him for the award. The following words are Carolyn's portrait of this respected business consultant, father of five, choir member and Christian leader:

I recall my first luncheon meeting with Hal. He was dressed very professionally and his speech was slow and deliberate. Each word was carefully planned out as if he had an agenda for this luncheon similar to a board meeting presentation.

Prior to his stroke, Hal was the chief executive officer of a company. He planned to eventually return to this position. He looked me straight in the eye and in a kind, gentle, aphasic voice told me that he would get his speech back some day. He had already proved the doctors wrong once by surviving his stroke. I could only respond, "Mr. Lance, you can do anything you put your mind to."

A perfect example of his determination was demonstrated when he asked me to sit in on a performance he was doing for his music enrichment class. Previously, a soloist in his church choir, Hal was now taking voice lessons. He had decided to do a solo presentation for the entire class.

Not wanting to make him uncomfortable, I stood behind closed doors and listened to him sing. When the piano began playing, I held my breath in anticipation of what kind of strained, unintelligible sound would be filling the room. He began singing, "You'll Never Walk Alone." To my surprise, through the poetry and rhythm of the music he uttered every word beautifully. Tears began to well up in my eyes at the magic this song held for Hal. All of his energy poured into each word. "You'll Never Walk Alone" expressed the essence of how Hal lives each day.

Hal is a sincere and gentle man who always focuses on the positive. He spoke to me about his six-year-old daughter and how he participated with her in an Indian Princess program. A father of five children, he has seen his stroke as an opportunity to become closer to his youngest daughter. Hal's office at home is a room filled with hopes and dreams. A photo of a broad-jumper at the Olympic trials hangs on the wall, a portrait of Hal in his earlier days. He has been able to use this office for a series of part-time, home-based job opportunities.

Currently, Hal is employed in logistics planning at the Pillsbury Company, Minneapolis, Minnesota. He is involved in future planning for various products and works on specialized projects with the aid of his home computer, but meets one afternoon a week with a team of individuals at Pillsbury. Hal also is a consultant for small businesses and is involved with projects such as mailing, financial planning and other business planning.

In a session delivered at the 1987 Stroke Seminar Hal summarized his philosophy: "When you feel like giving up, don't. If it hadn't been for my family and friends counting on me, I wouldn't be where I am right now. You can't give up; just keep going because they won't give up on you. You never walk alone."

from the Stroke Connection January 1983

How Bad Was Your Stroke?!

by Judy Hopia, Maple Plain, Minnesota

Last Tuesday someone asked me, "How bad was your stroke?"

I told them that ten years ago at Christmas I was in a wheelchair and my doctors had told my family that I might be living with a wheelchair for the rest of my life. They told my family, "Just be glad she's alive; you almost lost her." From intensive care to a wheelchair was a transition we were all so very grateful for. We thanked God for such a gift.

The following Thursday I met a young man who just recently suffered a stroke. I watched him with painful memories as he walked with his walker cane. He noticed me watching him, so I smiled and asked if he had had a stroke. "Yes, my left side is affected," he said.

I told him my obvious physical limitations were the same as his about 9 1/2 years ago. His eyes beamed while we talked. Then upon parting he said, "You have given me so much hope. I hope that ten years from now..." I pray for him that ten years from now...

In the eyes of that young man, I looked like the image of health.

My physical recovery has been fantastic. The limitations I have to live with almost cannot be noticed now. But life for me is a daily struggle just as it was ten years ago when I was in a wheelchair. It is only relative to the years and where I am with my residuals today.

The emotional pain of my loss is with me daily. I was a 25-year-old woman whom friends and family called "superwoman." I had an unbelievable amount of energy and goals. I could do almost anything, and I did it well. I was really going places!

The other day I visited with a 27-year-old woman who had a stroke in July. Earlier when we talked on the phone, I told her about the stroke groups organized around the state. I told her how we support and listen and try to help each other, how we have fun together, learn about each others' trials and accomplishments, and learn more through speakers and films about stroke and adjusting to the changes in our lives.

She hesitated to come into a group atmosphere because her physical recovery had been seemingly good, and because she might feel out of place, but she still felt she needed to talk to someone who could relate with her. I agreed to visit her later in the week, and upon meeting her at the door she appeared to be the image of health.

After talking with her for some time on a superficial level, I realized, when we got around to talking about our strokes, that I did not have to ask her how bad her stroke was. The pain she was living with was written across her face and flowed forth with the tears she unsuccessfully fought back. It is all so relative; *she had a very bad stroke!*

No, I did not see her having to use a wheelchair or a cane; her speech seemed as good as mine. She informed me that it had all come back within a few weeks.

She had just given her children lunch and was trying to clean up the mess, and I noticed that she was experiencing a great deal of frustration trying to do this. The children were ready for naps, the phone was ringing, and I had just arrived.

For most mothers 27 years of age this would be a normal day, the frustration level would be average and coping would not be so difficult. But since suffering a stroke eight weeks ago, she felt devastated.

She confided in me that she felt like a broken woman, not needed, not whole. She talked about the pain of the loss, the change in her body and personality, and the humiliation involved with these changes.

I could not see the residual she was talking about, the numbness and thalamic pain she was living with, the loss of energy and memory, or the generalized confusion.

My heart went out to her. I wanted to hold her and bear her pain for awhile, to say that everything would be OK, that all of this was just a bad dream and that tomorrow she'd wake up to find the nightmare over.

I gave her very little advice, although I may have magnified the hope (I know the reality of stroke and how there are differences in recoveries, how it's all so relative to each of us, and how our residuals are unique to each of us). I gave her my ear of compassion and understanding, my hand of comfort and my heart-filled prayers that she will find the strength for her recovery and life with stroke.

There are thousands of people experiencing a stroke every day. Many of these people do not have the appearance of having to live with stroke. Their residual is hidden from casual observation. The pain they and their families are living with is as bad as any other stroke. It is all relative to each of us.

Life after a stroke is very difficult, as we all know. As time goes on and our physical recovery looks better, it is difficult for our family, friends and society to understand the change in us; to understand why we act differently or find it impossible or frustrating to live within our old lifestyle and not be understood; not really being able to explain our residuals or even if we can, having someone look at us with disbelief because we look like we're recovered so well is defeating. Society's expectations of us are colored by what our recovery looks like or by what we look like we *should* be able to do. It's difficult to explain that maybe one day our energy level, frustration level, and our general being might seem good but then the next day we seem to fall back to day one with many of our residuals. I'm sure it's frustrating to them just as it is frustrating to us.

Whether we are in a wheelchair, or live in physical pain with no energy, whether we have lost the function of small and/or large motor nerves or have spasticity, whether we've lost our speech and communication functions with aphasia, or we have a field cut, whether we have lost our old learning or new learning has become difficult, we all have experienced stroke and know the pain involved with our own individuality.

We are fortunate to have each other through our stroke groups—

with a supporting network. We may not be able to explain and educate the outside world today about the experience of stroke; that may take some time. But we do have each other.

I'd like us all to try to be more broadminded with stroke and work on our compassion and empathy for each other. To keep in mind that each and every one of us has experienced stroke and the severity (bad stroke) is only relative and unique to ourselves. That the statement "How bad was your stroke?" is meaningless because all strokes can be devastating. We need each other. We all have our own pain to bear.

from the Stroke Connection February 1984

I Call You Friends
(John 15:15)

by Sister Winifred Edlebeck, Racine, Wisconsin

When we are strangers,
we need a friend who will
   smile at us
   welcome us
   call us by name.

When we are lonely,
we need a friend who will
   remember us
   visit us often
   cheer us.

When we are grieving,
we need a friend who will
   console us
   sustain us in grief
   be sensitive.

When we are insecure,
we need a friend who will
   reassure us
   listen to us
   show concern to us.

When we are happy,
we need a friend who will
   celebrate life with us
   thank God with us
   share our happiness.

When we are irritable,
we need a friend who will
   forgive us
   be patient with us
   overlook our complaints.

When we are dissatisfied,
we need a friend who will
   listen to us
   change conditions
   let us express our feelings.

When we are disturbed,
we need a friend who will
   calm our fears
   dispel our doubts
   bring peace of mind.

Editor's note: Sister Winifred Edlebeck, a Dominican sister and a stroke survivor, wrote the above reflection while she was a visitor for the homebound with the Senior Companion Program at Siena Center. She belongs to the Racine County Stroke Club, Wisconsin, and plays the piano.

from the Stroke Connection September/October 1988

In the Dreamtime

by Arthur Lusis, Seattle, Washington

I find it interesting that I should title my article about my stroke, "In the dreamtime," by borrowing the phrase, "the distant past," from the aborigines of Australia. Because that's the way it was.

It was in July of 1984 that I had two massive strokes at the ripe old age of 28. Suddenly, this apprentice bricklayer, who the day before was climbing all over an unfinished house, was dependent on everyone. One day I was in perfect health, and the next day I couldn't walk or use my left arm or hand, and the right side of my body felt like it had been dipped in copier fluid.

The prognosis was that I would remain in a wheelchair and would have to be taken care of the rest of my life. Boy was I mad. They pooh-poohed me when I told them that I would be walking within the month, because I was in denial. Darn right I was in denial. I didn't believe the prognosis for one second. Sure, I felt terrible and I looked terrible, but I felt that that kind of pronouncement should come from me, not someone else. In the first place, I was supposed to be dead—but I wasn't; they were wrong about my fate.

Almost four years later, I look normal, and I walk without the aid of any device. Now I'm the person I have always wanted to be, doing things without fear getting in the way. I will never want to go back to being the other "normal" that I was. At that time, I didn't have anything really going for me, except my health. I was doing a lot of self-destructive things then in search for the perennial "good time." Killing myself with kindness. I had no clue as to what life and inner happiness was all about. It took two strokes to wake me up.

Now I believe in myself. Now I know that the only thing that can get in the way is me. It was, indeed, knowledge almost worth dying for. As soon as you say you can't, you can't. The most satisfying event in my recovery is the use of my limbs; the second is in helping others similarly affected.

Oh, I still feel like my head is immersed in three-dimensional Jell-O. But hey, it will just take a little longer to do something, that's all. And if it doesn't, I can live with it. In my very short association with stroke, I've done things a lot of folks said wouldn't happen. I also know that I am very lucky to have been given the proverbial "second chance."

from the Stroke Connection June 1981

It's So Hard

by Bob Lepp, Courage Center, Golden Valley, Minnesota

*It's so hard to watch
her struggle while
she forms that single
half word.
What's she thinking about?
Does she want me to supply
the word for her? Will
she be mad if I do
or if I don't?
I don't like to see
her struggle.
It hurts me.
I don't like to see
her in pain.
She's already suffered
too much.
Can't I relieve some
of her struggle/pain/suffering?
It helps me to tell her I
care about her but
I can't make her stroke
go away. I can't make
her talk again.
Sometimes I wish I could go away
so I wouldn't have to watch.
I wish I didn't have to
watch her struggle.
For me watching her
struggle
is the worst part.*

from the Stroke Connection September/October 1988

Just the Way She Always Did for Me

by Jan Gerling, Minnetonka, Minnesota

When I was a child, my mother would often pay a surprise visit to my classroom. I recall the uncontrollable joy I would feel and wanted everyone to know this pretty lady was my mother. I'd say, "Hi Mom, come and see how clean my desk is inside." I loved things neat and orderly.

Then one day, my mother had a stroke. I, too, made frequent visits to the nursing home where she lived. Not expecting me, the look on her face was priceless as she spied me coming down the hall. She'd wheel her chair to me, give me a kiss and tell her friends, "She's my daughter, and I'm real proud of her." The strong fingers and hands that once braided and curled my hair became weak after her stroke. Now it was my turn to shampoo and set and style her silver hair.

Thinking back to her hospital stay, following the stroke, I remember how the roles suddenly reversed, and I became the mother. I stood over her and watched her sleep and doze, opening her eyes and closing them again. It's like she needed assurance that I was there. I pulled the sheet up over her shoulders, just the way she covered me as a child. I held cool wash cloths on her head to relieve the pain, just the way she did for me when I was hospitalized with a kidney infection. I spooned liquids into her feverish lips, the way she did for me when I was too small to remember.

I was with Mother when she had a seizure one night. I thought she was dying, but after it was over, she sat up and asked, "What happened?" I even slept in a chair beside her bed at night. She had done the same for my two brothers when they needed her in illness.

Mom was surrounded with love and prayers and showered with hugs, kisses and warm touches. Her pastor, neighbors, caring friends and concerned relatives all visited. My brother's little two-year-old would gently pat her face and say, "Gamma sick?"

Then the bad news came. "We've done all we can for your mother," the doctor said. "You must make arrangements for her care now. I can give you a list of nursing homes in your area if you'd like." I had to do something fast.

I decided to move her from Wisconsin to Minnesota just 10 minutes from my home instead of three hours one way. I packed up all of Mom's belongings, loaded her into the back seat of the car and off we went. I wondered to myself how many times she must have packed up diaper bags, clothes, water, pillows and potty chairs for us when we took family trips.

Mom was frightened when we arrived and hung on to me the same way I once clung to her skirt, screaming my head off on that first day of kindergarten. She cried, "Don't leave me."

Mom worked daily with therapists until she gradually learned to walk and talk quite well again. I spent hours going over her flash cards with her, just the way she did for me when I was learning my multiplication tables.

I remember the very first time I bathed my new baby daughter and how she cried. My mother lovingly gave her a small stocking to hold on to, and she calmed right down. She said, "Babies are afraid they are going to fall and feel more secure if they have something in their hand."

In the nursing home, Mom was frightened of the electronic chair lift that would raise her in the air before lowering her into the bathtub, and she'd reach out for my hand and say, "I'm scared." As if I were the mother I'd say "I'm going to stay right with you." I bathed my mother's body many times, scrubbed her back, washed her hair, wrapped her in warm towels, powdered her "buns" and put lotion on her arms and legs, telling her how good she smelled. (All reminiscent of when I was a little girl.)

Mom entertained everyone at the nursing home when she was regaining her speech. She'd laugh at herself, too, when the words wouldn't come out quite right. For example: "It was so hot in my room last night that I woke up in a pool of prostitution." When somebody talked about having their baby circumcised she said, "They should never simonize boys without anesthetic."

Laughter truly is one of the best medicines. It gives the muscles of the face, chest and belly a gently workout—like internal jogging. It lowers the pulse rate and blood pressure and is a universal language which makes people feel closer to one another. Laughter makes you feel refreshed, rejuvenated and replenished. It also heals.

I love stories with happy endings, and I'm proud of how well Mom did at the nursing home in just four short months. With her stubbornness, great sense of humor, strong determination and good Irish blood, she helped in her own miraculous recovery.

Today my mother is living independently and once again bathing herself, doing her hair, eating without assistance, writing in her journal and dialing her own phone numbers. She has a very comfortable elder-care apartment where children come to sing and entertain regularly, and where animals are brought in for some loving from the senior citizens. There are birthday parties, games, exercise classes, good meals and weekly church services. I praise God that she is able to be on her own again.

I am thankful to God for answered prayer, for good friends and neighbors, for caring church members and for her pastor who makes "house calls."

Clara Speer has written a poem titled—MOTHER:

> *I think it was a girlish hand, unlined,*
> *well tended when it held*
> *at first, my clinging baby hand in*
> *gentle grasp by love impelled.*
>
> *I think it was a youthful face that*
> *bent above me as I lay asleep,*

bright the eyes that watched my rest,
in that forgotten day.

I think it was a slender form
that bore my weight on tiring arm,
and swift young feet that watched my steps
to guide them from the ways of harm.

But years and cares have changed that form,
and face and hand have streaked with gray the hair;
yet is the heart as full of love
as in that other day.

And she has her reward; not fame,
or baubles bought in any mart,
but motherhood's brave crown,
the love and homage of her own child's heart.

from the Stroke Connection January/February 1987

Letting Go

by Alice Beer, St. Paul, Minnesota

It was very difficult for me to leave my paraplegic husband unattended for short periods of time when I became a caregiver for him. For some reason or other, I established rules for myself when I started caring for him at home. At the top of the list of rules was that I would never, ever leave the house when there would be no one with him. No one ever expected, nor did he demand, that I would be ever-present and waiting on every beck and call. It was I who would feel terribly uneasy when I needed to run to the bank or to the grocery store. A feeling of guilt would often accompany my anxieties.

My husband has been home now for more than two years since his last stroke. In this time, especially recently, I have learned so many things. I know now that he, too, needs time alone, all to himself. He even seems happy to bade me "good-bye" on occasion when I spend a morning away at a committee meeting. I realize now that he actually had been denied the opportunity to demonstrate his ability to manage alone. Since he has aphasia, he can't tell me, but his smile on my return tells it all!

My "letting go" has helped us both. It has proven that even though his handicap requires much care, the need for him to be left in quiet surroundings and to himself is very important too. For me, my "letting go" has given me a little freedom that is so restful, so restorative.

My "letting go" has resulted in a more contented and pleasant household. Last, but not least, I am a less anxious and less apprehensive caregiver!

from the Stroke Connection November 1987

Living on the Edge

by Jim Meier, Lake Elmo, Minnesota

Over the last few months, Marion Rasmussen, editor and chairperson of the *Stroke Connection*, has asked me several times about my being afraid of having another stroke, and how I cope with that fear. That question is often asked by others. This is my response to Marion's question, which I hope will offer some encouragement for others who are "living on the edge" like myself.

Statistics show that there is a 30 percent chance of a second stroke during the first year of recovery. But, after the first year, the long term outlook is 70 percent better than it was 30 years ago. Another positive statistic shows that the incidence of primary intracerebral hemorrhage has steadily declined since the mid-1940's. That sounds good doesn't it? But, a not so positive statistic shows that there has been no decrease in the incidence of subarachnoid hemorrhage.

In 1973, when I started taking medication, my doctor told me that if my blood pressure remained high, I probably could have serious health problems, even a hemorrhage. It never occurred to me, probably because I didn't listen very well, that I would ever have a hemorrhage. At that time I thought, "Hemorrhage? Me? Impossible!" I don't think that way any more. I've learned much about hemorrhage—the hard way. My stroke was caused by a brain hemorrhage in June of 1983; I was 44. The doctors found that I had two aneurysms in the subarachnoid area of the brain. The one on the left side had hemorrhaged and required immediate surgery. The aneurysm on the right side had not hemorrhaged and they elected not to operate yet on that side until they saw the results of the surgery on the first aneurysm.

This is the good news-bad news part of the story. My wife knew on the morning of the surgery, that it was going to be a long day. The good news was that at noon she was notified that the surgery had been completed, that it worked, and that I would be in postoperative recovery most of the afternoon. My wife must have relaxed after hearing that. But, the bad news was that later that day, at about

5:00, my wife was asked to come into the recovery room and to try to help calm me down because I was thrashing on the bed, pulling at tubes, and not communicating very well. I had had another stroke and, as a result, I had become aphasic. The doctors decided that it was too risky to operate on the other side of the brain. That is why I am living "on the edge."

I spent the next six months in primary recovery, mostly in speech therapy. During that time, I was angry and depressed, and I thought a lot about who and what I was, and what the type of future was ahead of me. My typical day was to sleep late in the morning, eat lunch which my wife prepared and then spend the afternoon watching T.V., or sit outside and look with an open stare at nothing. On the positive side, relatives and friends often stopped to say "hello" and ask how things were going. Those visits helped me erase some of the anger and depression.

It was quite a blow to me to be aphasic. Throughout my life I have worked in communications, either as a teacher or as a writer. My first efforts after the stroke were dismal. I couldn't read a newspaper; when I tried to write, my sentences were very short; and there was no continuation in thought—pure sub-elementary. When I went to bed at night, I often cried. My plea to God was usually, "Why me, why me?" and, "I'm sorry, I'm sorry, I'm sorry."

Fortunately (miraculously), with a lot of help, I was able to regain most of what I had lost. Six months after the stroke the doctors allowed me to go back to work. It's been four and one-half years since the hemorrhage, and most of the pain has softened. I feel that I'm probably a better person than I was before, but I still grieve for the loss of a part of me (stroke survivors know what that means). I know that I have an aneurysm on the right side of my brain, and I know that it would be too risky to try to correct the problem through surgery. I also know that if the aneurysm would hemorrhage, the prognosis would not be good at all. The question is—How do I cope?

I am from a very large family (six sisters, eight brothers), and I am the youngest. I have experienced many personal, excruciating losses. In 1949, my mother, age 53, died from her third stroke, I was eleven at the time. When I was 17, my father, age 59, died from a heart attack two weeks before I graduated from high school. It took me years before I could accept what happened to my parents. Since then, I have lost a brother, age 53, who died from a brain tumor; a sister, age 53, who died while having an angiogram; a sister who has diabetes, and who has lost three of her children through stroke-related problems. I have a sister who has had a heart attack; a brother, a sister, and a nephew who have had strokes; a brother, who has had a triple bypass; and a brother who has diabetes, and who recently had a angioplasty. I have learned to cope with losses—I had to.

There's no point trying to hide the risk or trying to gloss over what might happen. It's better to face the possibility of another stroke, resolve the issue, accept it, and then get on with life. In the old days, I used to live my life as if I were playing poker. That's a very chancy game, where the player hopes to get the right cards to win the pot. I don't bet or play games with life anymore.

Instead:
- I control my blood pressure.
- I carefully watch my diet.
- I avoid physical exertion.
- I use a mental stress exercise.
- I schedule walks.
- I laugh, whenever possible.
- I share love, and counsel with others.
- I enjoy my hobbies.
- I pray.

There are priorities on this list. If I were put to a test, I would put the bottom line, **pray**, at the top of the list. It's hard for me to respond to Marion's question. It's easier for me to simply raise my hands and shake my head with no answer. But, that's where the word **courage** comes in. Stroke survivors must continue, must be persistent, must be determined, and must not quit. I am afraid of what might, or might not happen during the rest of my life, but I cherish the good times and accept the not-so-good times. To answer Marion's question—I feel that this life was never meant to be perfect; but sometimes, I see a glimpse of how wonderful it will be when I am face-to-face with God. That's how I cope with "living on the edge." I pray that others have the strength and courage to do the same.

from the Stroke Connection August 1988

Man's Best Friend in Twilight Zone

by Mary (Mitzie) Childs, St. Louis Park, Minnesota

After spending months in the hospital after my stroke, I came home and had my son escort me to my bench in the backyard for some fresh air. I assured him I'd be okay and encouraged him to leave for awhile. With my dog, Dolly, and my daughter's dog, Davina, by my side, I was enjoying myself.

Suddenly, the fear of total abandonment took over my thoughts. "Is someone going to come and injure me? Oh, why did I tell my son to leave me alone?" The few minutes I was out there seemed hours. "When is he coming back?" My mind was clouded with every imaginable fear at this point. With some hesitancy, I grabbed my cane and decided to check out some trees.

I soon found out how disoriented I had become. I couldn't find my house (only a few feet away) and I studied a neighbor's home. I knew I lived next door someplace, but where? Oh, what a "Twilight Zone!" In desperation, I searched for my house. Apparently, the dogs sensed my fear and panic and began circling around me and barking wildly. I tried to see if anyone was near (my vision has become one of my deficits). They kept herding me until I was at my back door.

I crawled up the steps. Fearing the dogs would knock me down, I propped the door open with my cane, instructing them to go down into the basement. I knew I had more steps to climb to the kitchen. I crawled up there, sat on the floor and cried and cried. The dogs came to me, tails wagging. They knew they did a great job! I was so happy to be in my house after the traumatic experience.

from the Stroke Connection September/October 1987

Meeting a Challenge:
Dealing with My Stroke as an Adult Child of an Alcoholic Parent

by Jane A.

I survived a massive stroke eight years ago. I am still recovering physically, emotionally, mentally and socially from damage resulting from the stroke.

I have also survived growing up with an alcoholic mother. Her alcoholism was serious (she died from this disease). The effects on me of her alcoholism made my recovery from stroke more difficult in some ways than it may be for others who are not children of alcoholics. Some of the problems I have had are with:

- Denial
- Guilt
- Not asking for help
- Perfectionism

■ *DENIAL.* I have been accustomed since childhood to deny that problems exist, even very obvious ones, and to deny that I have any feelings about these problems.

Denial after stroke can be useful in the early stages, enabling some people to work harder because they believe they can do what they did before. As a continuing pattern, denial is harmful because it encourages a survivor to ignore the reality of the situation and the need to adjust to it. In my denial, I believed all along that I would be able to do almost everything I did before my stroke.

I did—and still often do—expect myself to be able to do things I would never expect of another person in my situation.

Denial like this led me to lowered self-esteem when I encountered my limits, anger at others for not taking care of the things I really could not do, exhaustion and depression.

My denial has included denying the losses to me that resulted from my stroke and denying the pain of these losses.

■ *GUILT.* Guilt is a feeling familiar to adult children of alcoholics. It begins with the child's belief that he or she is responsible for what is wrong in the family. Just as children of divorced parents typically blame themselves for the break-up, so do children of alcoholics believe that if only they were good enough, mother or father wouldn't have to drink. The fact that the disease of the parent often exists before the child did is sometimes, as in my case, not known until the parent dies.

Guilt after stroke seems common among stroke survivors I have met.

I knew very well all along that my stroke was not my fault, but I certainly felt guilty about the changes that my family experienced as the result of my stroke. In my case, I expressed to my family that feeling of guilt often enough, both directly and indirectly, that I believe they began to agree with me and to feel that they were the victims of my stroke.

I felt more guilt as I came to discover that my physical recovery would not be complete. Perhaps I had not worked hard enough on my therapy and exercises or transferring my therapy to daily chores. My guilt increased when I encountered others who had regained more use of the affected hand or whose walk seemed graceful and easy.

I know now that I really did the best I could all along. My partial recovery is a triumph—won through great effort, despite the fatigue and discouragement that were also a part of my stroke damage.

■ *NOT ASKING FOR HELP.* When an alcoholic parent is asked for help, it is rarely given. Soon the child learns not to ask in order to avoid disappointment. With lowered expectations, the child sees himself or herself as not worthy of help from others. "If you want something done, do it yourself" becomes the motto.

Not asking for help after stroke. With a lifetime of not asking for help behind me, I found it difficult, even in the hospital, to ask for what I needed. I think now of the embarrassment I felt when I didn't want to bother the nurses in the days before I regained bladder control. I did not ask for help. I remember a time when I could not eat a meal I wanted because I was too embarrassed to ask my visitors to cut the meat for me. I did not ask for help.

Becoming helpless in some of these ways has taught me that I can ask for help and that people are almost always delighted to give it —just as I am when I can help someone else. Learning that I am a person who can ask for, accept and give help has been an important process and a real source of joy to me.

■ *PERFECTIONISM.* Children who grow up in alcoholic family systems try hard to create some kind of order in the midst of chaos in order to lower their constant level of fear. I have heard this fear explained this way and I know it was true for me. The alcoholic parent is out of control; the other parent is unable to control the alcoholic; and these two people are in charge of the child. Small wonder the child tries to control every single thing in the environment that he or she can. My alcoholic mother never stopped being a perfectionist about a wide variety of things, even long after she was unable to do anything but drink! I learned early that only by doing things perfectly (i.e, her way) could I hope to get any approval from her.

Perfectionism after stroke. By the time of my stroke at age 39, I was not satisfied with anything I did unless it came close to my high standards. When I could not stand, or walk, or even sit up without falling to one side, I was disgusted with my inability to do the most basic things. My very patient and accepting therapists were able to encourage me and show me that I was making progress that I couldn't detect. It was very easy to please them, and I got daily expressions of approval.

I have finally learned that even though I don't do anything perfectly anymore, I am not responsible for the outcome, only for my efforts.

These four characteristic behaviors made my progress in recovery more difficult. However they were all things that I needed to acknowledge and work on as I struggle for recovery in my Adult Children of Alcoholic Al-Anon Program. It also seems that growing up in an alcoholic family system has been valuable training in learning some survival skills for dealing with other difficult life events.

It occurs to me that many of us—not just children of alcoholics—have these same behavior characteristics as a result of growing up in our culture where it is socially acceptable to deny pain, to feel guilty about things we didn't do, to be able to give but not ask for help from others, and to be perfectionists.

I feel that my stroke recovery has been enhanced by my working on these behaviors as part of my Al-Anon Program. I am finding that I feel much more comfortable with myself and my disability.

from the Stroke Connection March 1982

Misspellings

by Kristen Naylor

I can't spell

apple,

bicycle,

or gastroenterologist.

But,

I am trying.

Someday

-maybe-

and maybe

not.

from the Stroke Connection March 1988

My Sister Had a Stroke

by John T. Skalet, Evergreen, Colorado

In January 1982, my wife and I and our three-year-old son were visiting my wife's parents in Poughkeepsie, New York. It was an emotional time as my mother-in-law was undergoing radiation treatment for cancer.

My wife wished she had one of my mother's recipes with her, so I called my mother in Minneapolis, Minnesota. When she answered, I knew right away something was wrong. She said that she and my father had just received a call from Conrad, my sister's husband, who said Mary, my sister, was failing rapidly at Methodist Hospital after apparently suffering from a severe migraine; that she may die and that we had better get over there right away.

A feeling of panic came over me. How could I get there right away? How would Mary's six-year-old daughter, Laura, deal with this? How would my aging parents survive the loss of their only daughter? I just fell apart. It was one of those times when one finally realizes how much someone means to you. You feel like it may be too late for them to ever know how you felt. She had been swimming at Northwest Athletic Club and had become disoriented and was not coming to the surface. Fortunately, a paramedic and his vehicle were at the club. He pulled Mary from the pool and rushed her to the hospital.

The physician on call was concerned over Mary's partial consciousness and admitted her to intensive care for observation. His action saved Mary's life. At that point, no one except the doctor realized the seriousness of her condition. Mary's condition deteriorated from that point on—apparently caused by the swelling of her brain, the buildup of fluid and reduction of blood flow to the brain. Neurologists had been called and were watching closely with brain scan equipment. Nearly 24 hours after her stroke, Mary went from unconsciousness to almost not breathing. If she would not have been in intensive care, she would have died. A shunt was put into Mary's skull to relieve the pressure, a move that without question saved her life.

This event began an emotional roller coaster for our family and friends. After a week with Mary at the hospital, I needed to return to work in Denver. Mary had not improved at all. She lay in a shuffling unconsciousness, connected to about 20 tubes and a respirator to force her to breathe. I felt the continual awareness that without all that life support, my sister would be dead. Still, I was concerned about the ability of my parents, Conrad and Laura to handle the situation. Was this really happening to my family and my sister? I felt so empty returning to Denver. My mother seemed to assume most of the burden.

As the weeks went by, we talked by phone each night—sometimes twice—sometimes in the morning, too. I tried to reassure her. There was so little change when we talked that we weren't even sure which direction Mary was heading. About two weeks after Mary's stroke, the doctors attempted to remove the shunt and it broke off inside Mary's skull. We felt a sense of panic. Why did this happen? What will they do? How will it affect Mary's recovery? Specialists were called in and the shunt was removed. Before the surgery, Mary had just begun to react to others. Now she went back into almost total unconsciousness for nearly a week.

The burden on my mother spending each day with her was really taking it's toll. I tried my best to prop my mother back up at the end of each day but the drain was tremendous. Progress continued to be almost nil. The weeks went by. The real breakthroughs were, "She made a sound." "She seemed to understand." "She swallowed some Jell-O." "She hates the catheter." What we saw of Mary's returning personality only made us all realize that the person coming back was not the same Mary. Her stroke had made her very paranoid and she was short with everyone. It scared us—would we ever have our Mary back?

I planned a trip back to Minneapolis about six weeks after Mary's stroke. I had not been able to witness first-hand any improvement being so far away. It was a special time for Mary and me. We felt a closeness we had never experienced before. I think Mary had some desire to show me that she was going to beat her disability. We talked so much about how we both felt. Others told me that it was the first time she had done much talking at all. I wheeled her to the sun room for the first time and, oh my, was she dizzy, but happy for a moment.

One day she told me she needed to have the nurse bring her a bed pan but I said that I thought she could handle it if I could walk her to the bathroom. She seemed scared but challenged. She said "Do you think we could?" I said, "Sure!" First we sat together on the side of the bed and then stood up together, hanging on to each other. The look on her face was that of a nine-month old standing up for the first time at the side of the coffee table. We took cautious steps to the bathroom and I placed her down on the toilet. She called me when she was ready and we walked back to the side of her bed. She was so pleased, I was so pleased, an experience that I will never forget as long as I live.

Mary improved significantly over the next few weeks and was released from the hospital several weeks later. She had improved so much that by June, six months later, she flew to Denver with Laura, her daughter, for a visit. As she staggered out of the plane like a drunk, under her own power, the tears rolled down my cheeks. I tried to hold them back because I didn't want her to think I was ashamed. I actually was proud, so proud of my sister, a survivor. I felt as though she had won.

I had no awareness of how difficult the years ahead would be, especially for her, having to be a person with a different personality and unable to do the things she had been so good at before. Today, almost six years later, those who know her see her as nearly 100 percent recovered. Those very close to her know that she is still not all the way back, but she's gaining. If I know my sister, she will continue to gain for the rest of her life, and she will be a better person from the experience.

from the Stroke Connection November 1982

My Definition of Acceptance

by Jane Anderson, Minneapolis, Minnesota

"Don't be such a Pollyanna," we want to say to people who claim to see a silver lining around misfortune. I used to think people who talked about accepting a stroke were all Pollyannas. Usually, they were people who were not disabled by stroke; how could they possibly understand? Adjusting, maybe. Adapting, one has to. But accepting all the changes after a stroke? How, Pollyanna?!

Acceptance has come to have many meanings to people who have experienced stroke. I'd like to share mine. I like it; I worked hard to find it; and it has given me a lot of comfort through a long stretch of hard times.

For a long time, the idea of accepting such an awful catastrophe as stroke seemed really bizarre to me. I figured if I could *adjust* to living with disability I would be doing the most I could. Art Greenough of the Minneapolis Stroke Club, over lunch in the Courage Center cafeteria one day, started me thinking further about it. Then I couldn't *stop* thinking about what acceptance might mean in my terms. Thank you, Art.

I was on shaky ground to begin with. Not only had I not yet adjusted to my disability, I had never really developed much acceptance of myself as a person before my stroke. You see, I think accepting who you are, as a disabled person, means you need to be able to accept yourself as a person, first. Who you are—what is unique about you— does not change because of the sudden onset of disability. The "old me" and the "new me" are the same in all important aspects. Who you are means your personality, your likes and dislikes, your own brand of tastes and sense of humor (or lack of them), your talents, your personal memories, your particular history. A continuing sense of identity over time is a priceless asset.

Who you are is *not* an arm and a leg, and it's absurd to think of yourself that way—others don't. People who care about you don't pay much attention to your warts—your wrinkles, your faults. They care about the person inside, not the wrapping. So accepting yourself as a disabled person means accepting yourself, who you are inside. My family showed me all about it by refusing to be embarrassed by my disability.

Acceptance may require that you repeat to yourself, as some have suggested, "I'm OK just the way I am—I'm good enough (for today) the way I am." Believing that takes a lot of effort and proving to yourself that you are as close as you can come (for today) to satisfying your worst critic—yourself.

But acceptance is kind of like housework—it won't stay done. It's hard to be different. Acceptance often gets pushed behind more pressing feelings (anger, frustration, loneliness, etc.) and needs to be taken out again and polished up for further service. It's like insurance to know you have it when you need it most. Sometimes a friend will remind you that "you need it, too." Stroke club friends are great at showing us the need to reaffirm our acceptance.

I wish I could bottle acceptance and share it with you—but acceptance is something we each have to develop in our own way, when we're ready. For many, it is based on belief in God—turning over our troubles to God can help us accept them. For some, our problems can be seen as a gift from God, to prove we are worthy of a trial.

The Protestant theologian and philosopher, Paul Tillich, helped me to get to acceptance of stroke in an essay, not about disability but about our fundamental separation from God through sin. He speaks of "accepting the unacceptable" in a book with a beautiful title, *The Courage to Be*. He talks about "the courage to be as oneself" defined as "the courage to make of oneself what one wants to be." I thought about these phrases for weeks and emerged with my acceptance.

Another source for me was the writings of Flannery O'Connor, a brilliant young writer disabled by lupus erythematosus. Her route to acceptance took many years of working and renewing. A dear friend of hers wrote about O'Connor "making the most of her gifts and her circumstances"—and I think this is the essence of how her acceptance helped her.

All right, I'm not OK—as OK as I once was—and I don't have to like what's happened to me. I'd like to get better, and I still believe I will.

from the Stroke Connection November/December 1983

Odyssey

by Inez Thoren, Buffalo, Minnesota

7:30 a.m. I stuff my sandwich into my purse, check the stove and kiss my spouse "good-bye" as I rush off to another routine day of work. Routine? That's what I thought. But—I come home to find my house in a turmoil. Neighbors are there; several big men I've never seen before are in my living room; and there's an ominous-looking truck parked in front of the house. What's up? Is my house on fire? No. The cause is much more devastating and permanent than a fire. My husband has had a stroke. The rescue squad is waiting for the ambulance and I try to piece together what has happened. But my husband can tell me nothing. He is unable to speak except for a few garbled words which are meaningless. The ambulance arrives and I climb into the cab for the trip to the emergency ward, too stunned to sort out the implications of what has happened. But somehow I know—I just know—that life will never be the same again.

Through the long hours which stretch into days, weeks and months, I somehow move through the maze of tests, brain surgery, paralysis, tracheotomy and waiting. Finally, there is partial recovery, rehabilitation with physical therapy, occupational therapy and speech therapy. With further recovery and the prospect of eventual discharge, my own apprehension increases. How will I manage when he comes home? How will I cope with his disability and especially, lack of communication? Will he be happy to be home or will he resent the limitations of his handicaps? How will he respond to my making all the decisions and assuming the activities he once took for granted as his prerogatives? How does a brain-damaged mind work, and how can I know what he thinks? Oh, there are so many questions! Where can I turn for answers, and how have others in similar circumstances coped with the problems that now confront me?

My first source of information was the public library. I took out every book I could find, some of them twice, which gave me some answers to my questions. Then, fortunately, I heard about stroke clubs. An announcement in the local paper invited anyone interested in such a group to a meeting at the library, and thus the Wright County Stroke Club was born. This fledgling group, with no funding and little support, was my ray of hope. I knew that a club could not make my husband less aphasic or more alert or stronger physically. But here were people—wonderful, caring, dear people—who understood what my problems were. They, too, were seeking to put the pieces of their lives together again. They, too, knew the joys of small successes, as well as the heartache of continued failures in the long journey to a more meaningful and normal life. We were not alone! Here are friends—people who do not shy away from us because they are uncomfortable trying to communicate with us. They have experienced, in varying degrees, the same anxieties, frustrations, anger, hopes and despair we have. Here are people who can truly share our feelings when we are "down" as well as the elation of victory when progress, however small, is made. We see others who are even less fortunate than we are and it makes us thankful. We see the accomplishments of those who have worked hard and long to make it to where they are, and it inspires patience. We see the cheerfulness and courage of those whose lives have been devastated in a manner similar to ours, and it gives us hope.

On one day of the month, we look forward to seeing and being with these gallant people. Oh yes, the wide variety of the programs makes it interesting, informative, inspiring and entertaining. But it is the people who draw us to this group—we see the warmth of their smiles when we greet them, to feel the squeeze of a hand and know the empathy and love which prompt it, to share a small moment of triumph in our own or someone else's odyssey—this is what makes stroke club the supportive and helpful occasion that makes that special day on our calendar each month. Blessings on stroke clubs!

from the Stroke Connection April 1986

One Step at a Time

by Dorothy Trollen, Red Wing, Minnesota

Ten months ago, a right hemisphere stroke left me with a paralyzed left leg and arm. The hand and arm are still useless—they are more in the way than anything. But with a brace and much therapy, the leg is now functional. I can walk with a quad-cane. I look healthy enough, but heavy brain damage has left me with neurological problems. It may not seem a tragedy that an adult woman cannot dress herself, but it is demoralizing and adds to the stroke survivor's feelings of helplessness.

When my children come to take me for a winter outing, I feel like a three-year-old being stuffed into my coat, hat and mittens.

When Rick, our occupational therapist, gave me yet another dressing lesson this week, he found me only partially dressed and in tears. When I called myself "dumb" he insisted, "No! Do not say that. Your dressing problem has nothing to do with intelligence. It is caused by brain damage and a lack of ability to recognize processes like sequencing." Therefore, I once put a sweater on right over my nightgown. Today, Faye, a nurse's aide, was helping me dress. She asked me why I was taking off the sweater that she had painstakingly put on me. I had no sensation of doing this. I wonder if it has to do with a sense of direction.

Meantime, I keep working in therapy on perceptual motor tasks. I keep the faith that with time and work my normal abilities will return.

I have a snapshot of my granddaughter at age two, wearing a new sundress that I had gotten for her. She had the denim bloomers on her head. Now, I have great empathy for the two-year-old and her dilemma.

from the Stroke Connection May/June 1987

Our Young Family Changes Direction

by Mar Hylbak, Apple Valley, Minnesota

$\mathbf{M}$y life changed drastically one Christmas Eve five years ago. As we were about to embark on a move to Colorado, our lives came to a halt and our goals were completely changed.

My husband had a stroke, an aneurysm, while we were vacationing at my parents' home. Two brain surgeries, eye surgery, months of therapy, pain, frustration and devastation followed; the details are so similar in many respects to others we've read about. But what makes us different is that we are a young family. My husband was only 31 years old, my daughter three and a half years old, and my son, an infant only five months old. I recall trying to wean him while sitting in the intensive care unit wondering if he'll ever know his Dad.

Well, life certainly has changed, but one thing was well answered— he really does know his Dad. You see, even though Dad's recovery hasn't been complete enough to allow him to go back to work full-time, we've adjusted our goals and Luke, our son, has his own personal version of "Mr. Mom."

The five years that have lapsed have made our family look very different than what we had imagined. Being young and naive, we had very traditional roles planned. But when Steve had his stroke, I thought it never would progress to where we are today.

Slowly, but surely, Steve has been able to take over more responsibilities at home. It certainly is not what he would have chosen to do, but working full-time is not what I would have chosen either.

I guess that has been the answer for us. Our family has had to change directions. We were forced to turn a corner.

It's been challenging raising two preschoolers, going to graduate school, working full-time and helping my husband recover. The past five years have been blurred by constant activity and pressure. But as we all continue to march ahead, acceptance of our unique family structure finally seems to be settling in. All of the answers aren't here for us yet, but commitment and love is abundant.

Sometimes when I look too far in the future, I get scared. What if he never works full-time again? What if I get sick? When will our kids really understand what happened to Dad? Will we look back and be satisfied with our lives as we age?

But then I think back to what my father taught me at a very young age. Life has no guarantees. Not for anyone! Many families face similar struggles—stroke, death, divorce, chemical abuse. There are many families solving struggles and living non-traditionally.

We're doing the best we can. I know that! And as we look back, we work at focusing on the positive. We're working to solve our problems. But thankfully, we're still a family together.

from the Stroke Connection April 1988

Reaching for Tomorrow

by Jim Meier, Lake Elmo, Minnesota

*Yesterday I said good-by
to what I used to be,
and cut the inner thread I had,
to find another me.*

*I tried with hope to hold it,
and keep me as a one.
But didn't know the final stroke,
was soon to break my soul.*

*Yesterday, in a hopeless way,
I tried to touch my life.
But there was I without a wing,
a voice to sing, not me.*

*I was the helpless, crying clown,
who tried to make you laugh.
But had to play the empty lead,
with nothing for to see.*

*Yesterday I tried to walk,
and tried to sing and fly.
But there was I with
        a broken mind,
and a hopeless, inner me.*

*With nothing left I tried to turn,
to what I used to be.
But had to wave my broken wing,
at life I'll never see.*

*Yesterday, in a tortured way,
I slowly walked away.
But why? But why? said I, said I,
was I the reason why?*

*You gave me wings and
        a voice to sing,
and a hope to see tomorrow.
But now it's done and I am left,
with a broken wing and me.*

*Today I closed my inner door,
and opened up a maybe.
But what might come, as yet to be,
if only I could see.*

*With a broken wing, and
        a broken mind,
I walk into the night.
Reaching, reaching, reaching,
for tomorrow and my dream.*

from the Stroke Connection June 1985

Reflections on My Stroke

by Ruth Munson, Oakdale, Minnesota

We stroke survivors live in a very self-involved world. While we try to find ourselves, we lose sight of the fact that those around us are helpless and hurt when they cannot share our pain.

They do not stop caring about us after the initial phone calls and the cards, gifts and flowers have been sent. But they are busy with their own lives. We stroke survivors need to let them know that we still care about them. It only takes a moment to pick up the phone or send a few "hello" cards.

Opening ourselves up to our friends and dear ones is a healing process on the road back. We are the same people we were but must communicate that we want to reclaim as much as possible the best of what we have in ourselves.

I have retained my former friends and have made many new ones. So many have been kind to my husband and me, helping with tasks which I still have a hard time doing such as sewing and mending. I still like to entertain and I have a friend who comes in to assist us.

None of us realizes that, unlike most illnesses, after a stroke we may not heal quickly. None of us—patients, doctors or therapists—can know when or how much of our former selves we will regain. So we have to accept what we are through patience and perseverance, continuing to hope for ongoing progress in our endeavor to live as rich and involved a life as possible.

from the Stroke Connection February 1984

Since My Stroke

by Jeanette Weeks, Minneapolis, Minnesota

Since my stroke, I have had considerable time to reflect on the many changes and transitions that have occurred over the past several months. Initially, all I could feel was sadness for the lost "things" in my life which focused on body parts and brain functioning, such as memory, numbers, attention span, judgment and perception. Now, I have learned a lot about the loss of these "things" and I realize I felt sadness only because I valued these "things." However, now, almost one and a half years later, I have relearned many skills. Most importantly, I have had time to learn that my priorities in life are different than before my stroke.

I am still basically the same person; I am at times inconvenienced or disadvantaged by my deficits and disability. But I learned that in a way, having survived a stroke has been a positive experience in teaching me that my family and friends are more important to me than ever. I have learned humility and have capitalized on my sensitivity.

The entire experience has not always been positive, but I can redirect my life now and make it better than ever. Without having sustained a disability, I never would have discovered the new me.

from the Stroke Connection May 1983

Speech

by Kristen Naylor

> *I talked with words,*
> *and then,*
>   *suddenly*
> *I became . . .*
>   *silent.*
> *I was frightened,*
> *and so*
>   *alone.*
> *Thank God*
> *it came back to me.*

from the Stroke Connection September/October 1987

Stroke Awareness

by Gennie Barnett, Seattle, Washington

Trying to educate the public about stroke through the media will never have more than limited success. Society is so fast-paced that we tend to skim over anything that is not novel or is not of immediate practical value to us.

I am convinced that the best way to grab the attention of people is through the demonstrated competence of disabled people. Every successful blind person I meet enlarges my knowledge about the problems of the blind. The pity is that blind people tend to move in nonsighted circles. I am fascinated by sign language and always anxious to learn more about the deaf, but to do so I must seek them out on their own turf. I wonder, how visible are stroke people?

People are interested in winners. They are turned off by whining, self-pity, and self-dramatization. They are intrigued by success, especially when they can't figure out how it is managed! When strangers become aware that I live alone and don't have a car, I get asked a lot of personal questions: Can I take my own bath? Do my own hair? Cook? Shop for groceries and clothes?

We need men and women who exemplify the role of the successful stroke survivor in order to educate the public about stroke. We need stroke survivors who are leading active lives in the community, so that others may be aware of them.

Some years ago, I visited a large church and encountered all sorts of obstacles trying to make my way forward for communion. Eventually, I had to be assisted and was embarrassed by the commotion I had caused. When I later commented about it to a deacon, he informed me that the handicapped people in the congregation preferred to have the priest administer the sacraments to them at home. How sad!

We need to be reminded often that we are all one, with seen or unseen frailties.

from the Stroke Connection September 1982

Stroke *Victims???*

by Jane Anderson, Minneapolis, Minnesota

Are we stroke victims? Probably not. The dictionary defines a victim as one who is injured, destroyed, sacrificed, tricked or duped. If we have had a stroke, or if we care about someone who has had a stroke and we are hanging in there, we're not victims at all, but survivors.

It's time for us to realize that the language we use influences us and others in forming attitudes. Stereotypes (such as stroke victim) are usually negative ways of looking at a group of people as if they were all alike and not individuals. The words we use to define a group can lead to bias for or against that group. If we find ourselves at some time unexpectedly joining a group we have always despised, then we have some self-hatred to overcome. If, on the other hand, we join a group we have admired, our self-esteem rises with our identification with the group.

The use of a word like "victim" with its many negative connotations can hurt our self-esteem when it is used about us or about a group of people with whom we identify. Certainly, having a stroke injured us and continues to cause problems for us, but it does not necessarily follow that we all act like victims, passively allowing ourselves to be helpless, dependent and sorry for ourselves.

If we do see ourselves as victims, what does this mean for us? Perhaps it means that our future is totally out of our control. Through no fault of our own, our choices are limited by our disability. We must settle for less than what we want. We become bitter—and soon lonely, because people who are bitter do not make good company and find themselves without friends. This unhappy situation is the result of seeing ourselves as victims. On the other hand, when we see ourselves as survivors, we rethink our dreams to fit our reality and this helps strengthen our self-esteem. Instead of being weak and helpless, we see that we are capable of overcoming obstacles, of transcending limits, of accepting the unacceptable. We approach the life we were spared with a new joy, a fresh appreciation, and the confidence of winners—of survivors.

We *can* choose: Victim or survivor, misery or acceptance, love or loneliness.

from the Stroke Connection January 1986

Surviving the Changes

by Alice Beer, St. Paul, Minnesota

Life has changed and we continue to adapt. After we were home for a while—home from the nursing home—it seemed somehow that every room needed a kind of alteration. I hedged, but after a time realized that it would benefit my helper, my spouse and me. The first huge forfeiture was carpeting. The Hoyer lift just would not move its wheels on the plush paprika-colored carpeting in the master bedroom, Urban's room. I pulled and I tugged until I injured myself and was sorely in need of medical attention—an x-ray of my painful hip. The diagnosis was a pulled ligament. Only then, after spending some money unnecessarily and going without some much needed sleep—did I relent. I called the company that had laid the carpet only a few short years before. Yes, they would come the next day and, for a price, would remove the beautiful floor covering. They would roll it and store it in the attic. I'm reluctant to admit it, but can say truthfully that it has been smooth rolling ever since! Finding a shiny, hardwood floor, waxed and polished underneath, was a pleasant surprise. It's easy to maintain and keep clean with a dust mop and an occasional wet wipe. I wonder now why I struggled to keep things in that room as they were. I guess I wasn't ready at the time to subject myself to yet another change.

The kitchen was almost perfect. The floor covering had been replaced with new linoleum one year before my husband's stroke. However, the cottage curtain over the sink interfered with Urban's bird-watching. I loved those curtains and really did not want to remove them. After a time, however, the south-facing window had its curtain taken off! My reward was Urban's happiness in seeing the sky, the planes going over and, of course, the birds on the fence at the feeder. In time I found that two long planters with greenery on the sill decorated that window sufficiently. It didn't seem bare after a while. One adjusts!

On our little screen porch there were colorful director's chairs. They were inviting, but left no room to accommodate a wheelchair over the threshold. One of our helpers brought wood from an old door and built a short ramp at the stoop and the two chairs were taken to storage.

The dining table was always perfectly aligned so that the chandelier with crystal prisms was centered above it. Moving the dining table was not a major concession. It was moved to the side and two dining chairs had to be taken from one side. Now the wheelchair can glide by easily and isn't apt to gouge or scratch any furniture.

My husband spends most of the day in the den. We had mylar window shades installed all around. The sun's rays are deflected, there is no glare and we can still see the outdoors. We can see three streets from this vantage point. When people walk by and look up, no one can see us. Two upholstered chairs had to be moved to storage to make room near the windows for the wheelchair.

The living room needed few adaptations. Urban is no longer able to build fires, but we have compromised by using lighted candles behind the fireplace screen. The candles give an illusion of a fire and they are bright and cheery. We've spent many winter hours watching their flickering glow!

Last, but probably the most drastic change, happened to the front of our house. Its image is quite different from what it was. We needed a 32 foot ramp to accommodate the less than 5 degree slope. I consulted a contractor and was completely dissatisfied with what he had to offer. His plan would ruin the looks of our front entryway and lawn. After a while, I registered my complaints and concerns with our visiting public health nurse. She offered to check with someone at St. Paul Rehabilitation Center for us. After quite a lengthy wait, from April to August, they built a beautiful ramp. Just outside our front door, covering the old stone steps, is a 5 foot square deck. The ramp leads from there. It is painted to perfectly match the red trim on our tan stucco house. Urban is able to go outdoors now with very little help. It wasn't long though, before we realized that the needles of the two aging evergreen trees close by were creating a hazard as they cluttered the ramp. They stuck to the tires of the "four wheeler" and could make them slip and slide. You've guessed it! The huge pine trees were toppled one rainy day in spring—almost one year after the ramp had been planned and erected. I'm quite comfortable living without those big trees, but I never dreamed I could be.

These are some of the changes we made so that our home might be adapted to a handicapped person residing in it.

One rather difficult adjustment for me personally was that my room became a warehouse for surplus furniture. It has a very busy look with unmatched pieces. However, on many nights it has become a haven. There are evenings after busy days when weariness overtakes a stroke survivor's spouse.

from the Stroke Connection September 1985

Take Time to Look Back

by Marion Rasmussen, St. Paul, Minnesota

During the process of attaining our goals, we must occasionally look back to see how we are doing in reaching each goal and whether they are all still worth the effort.

In looking back, we are able to see whether we have strayed too far from our goal. Or we might realize that in working toward a particular goal we have obtained some strengths not apparent before.

When I was growing up, I heard very little about setting goals. In fact, I did not think much about setting goals until I entered a master's program and started a new career of teaching at age 50.

As I look back on my life, I now realize that I actually set goals but did not consciously recognize them. I suppose my first formal experience with goal setting was during the period of Lent. Candy, when I was a youngster, was a great treat, so giving it up for six weeks during Lent was in reality setting quite a goal. My three brothers and I would save our special goodies in separate boxes, hoarding and hiding them, safeguarding our hoard against snooping siblings. In those days, Lent ended at noon on Holy Saturday. During the lengthy Holy Saturday services, my thoughts turned often to the sweet treasure waiting for me at home. At noon we ate a "Sunday" dinner after which we children could devour our cache of candy. I never regarded abstaining from candy for six weeks as a goal, but rather as a penance, much as I regarded giving up smoking during Lent in later years.

Growing up in the '30s, a time of economic stress in our family, left little time for daydreaming or elaborate fantasies. In a one-parent family, my mother set the goals. We children did what she expected of us. There was love, fun and laughter—and tears, but there were no burning desires to be fulfilled. It was a time of austerity, a time of having only enough money to pay the mortgage and to pay for food. The goal for all of us was simply to survive.

I had passing fancies of being a dress designer or a dancer and, of course, a mother. What I was going to do until that glorious day when I became one, I did not even contemplate.

It was when I was in high school that I became enamored of a career in medicine. I wanted to be a psychiatrist. Economic circumstances had changed favorably, but my ambition was short-lived. My mother's admonitions, "Women don't become doctors," and, "A psychiatrist? All psychiatrists are crazy" left me with no career save the one she encouraged me to enter—that of being a medical records librarian. It was a new field, she felt, and one in which I would make money and possibly meet and marry a doctor. I would be set for life! Such innocent thinking, but really based on her desire for me to have a better life than she had. *Her* goal!

So I graduated, worked, married, had two children, made jam, cooked and cleaned, until my older daughter was a sophomore in high school. Then I formally set a goal (but I did not think of it as a goal), to earn money to help my children through college. Eventually, ambition became a burning desire. I started out earning money teaching knitting and crocheting in a shop which led to my teaching those crafts in adult education, which led me to my desire to teach in my field. After 50 years, I had found my real goal— teaching.

I dived headfirst into a master's program, loved being called "Grandma" by some of the students, loved being part of the college life again, loved being immersed in study, loved being awakened again to philosophy and other academic subjects. I was accepted as an instructor in my field and taught for almost three years, with just a few credits left to finish my master's degree when my life came crashing down upon me. I had a stroke.

Then I learned the significance of goals and how important it is to set them.

Parallel bars, walk, Marion. Lift your right foot, Marion, lift your foot—your right foot. Now take a step. Raise your arm as high as possible, Marion, say your name. Say "thanks." Say "thanksgiving." Do you know what this word is? Do you know what the man is doing? Try to write that sentence. What does it mean? Say your name.

Take two steps. I'm walking with a walker. I'm walking with a tricane, I'm walking with a cane. Just as far as the next room. Just as far as the neighbor's steps. Just a few doors down. Half a block, one block, then around the block.

Read a sentence. Read a paragraph, read the article. Say nursery rhymes, sing nursery rhymes. Speak slowly. Think before you speak. Write the alphabet. Write a "d" and a "b."

Five months after my stroke I was writing thank-you notes in a childish, hesitant scrawl, copied from a master copy.

Each step I took, each letter of the alphabet I wrote, each phonetic sound I uttered was a goal achieved. A small goal, perhaps sometimes only a minute change in progress, but all together, these goals have brought me to where I am today—a disabled, able-bodied person.

It is only after we add the yesterdays to the yesterdays that the full magnitude of our progress can be measured. We cannot start at "A" and jump to "L" without first stopping at "B," "C" or "D" along the way. Each step has to be recognized as progress, however minor that step might be. Then, as we look back, we can recognize that we did something today that we could not do yesterday—raising a finger, taking a step, smiling at a friend.

Only in looking back was I able to realize how much I had recovered. In looking back, I also realized that I seldom think of my losses but more of my gains—gains that an "able-bodied" person would sniff at—but for me are significant benchmarks, a gain as insignificant as finally, after weeks or months of trying, remembering a friend's telephone number. For me, that's a gain.

Sometimes that gain is in reality a creative way of doing something in a different way. But that is still a gain. It is a progression.

The road to recovery is never easy. There were many roadblocks for me, many disheartening setbacks. I remember that road well but I need to look back occasionally to see how far I have come and how many small steps it took for me to walk that road back. At the same time, in looking back, I realized that I have set goals all my life, whether I realized it or not. In looking back I also realized that I remember mostly the gains or the goals I set for myself and for the most part those gains were happy occasions—occasions that are worthy to put in one's memory book.

from the Stroke Connection July/August 1984

The Four Keys to Living with Stroke

by Walt Collins, Mahtomedi, Minnesota

In May, I had the opportunity to speak to the Huron, South Dakota, Stroke Club and members from Sioux Falls and Aberdeen stroke clubs.

I told the groups a little about my background and my stroke, but my main message to stroke survivors and families was "how to live with stroke." My talk centered around four keys that open the doors to life after stroke.

■ The first key that unlocks the door to life is, "Once a person has had a stroke, that person is no longer the same person." Once the person accepts this fact, that person can go to the second key.

■ The second key to the door of life after stroke is, "Find out what kind of a person you are now." I think you might find out how much you like yourself.

■ The third key and, to me, the most important one is, "You have been given another chance at life. This time make it better."

■ The fourth and final key to the door of life is, "Relax—take time to smell the roses." I hurried through life before and look what I got—a stroke.

My hat is off to the wonderful people of South Dakota and especially to Stella Jennewein, president of the Huron Stroke Club. I had a most pleasant experience and they were most hospitable.

from the Stroke Connection November 1985

The ABC's of Coping with Disability

by Rosemary Froehle, MSW, Courage Center

A Acknowledge/accept what has happened in self and others

B Build support systems—professional, other people with similar disabilities

C Caregivers—take care of yourself

D Different is neither better nor worse, it's just different

E Emotional pain—acknowledge losses, but don't get lost in them

F Family and friends: stay in touch—***you*** contact ***them***

G Good grief—expressing sadness or sorrow is important and healthy

H Humor: don't take things too seriously, especially yourself

I Interest in others, life—keep learning

J Joy in simple pleasures: sunset, birds, children

K Know when to give in; know your own limitations

L Look at what you can do, not at what you can't do

M May not do same way, but still get job done doing it differently

N Nurture yourself—give to self in healthy ways

O One day at a time

P Patience and perseverance

Q Quit being perfectionistic, rigid

R Resources: Metro Mobility, adult day care, congregate dining, senior programs

S Self-image—change who am I—I'm still man or woman, a human being

T Tolerance of others who are different

U Use or lose it

V Visit others

W Wheelchair—it's liberation, not confinement

X "Xercise"—different ways

Y *You* are special, unique, important

Z Zest—keep it in your life.
Don't zip yourself out of life!

from the Stroke Connection November 1986

The Silent Explosion

by Walter Collins, Mahtomedi, Minnesota

Today, I would like to share with you some observations about my stroke as well as some of the learning experiences which brought new meaning to my life.

But before I do, a brief history of my stroke would help set the scene. My stroke occurred on July 8, 1981 at around 9:15 a.m. when a blood clot hit my brain. After a hospital stay of 10 days at St. Joseph's Hospital in St. Paul, my home became my recovery center. Therapy was important to the recovery of my left side, and I responded, not only during therapy three days a week at the hospital, but at home as well. Most homes have steps of some kind and I used mine for therapy. Also, my grandchildren's toys were adapted to use as occupational therapy equipment during my days at home.

About six months after my stroke, during one of my checkups, my doctor suggested that I visit a neuropsychologist. This was the best advice I have ever received. I believe that my recovery was much more rapid because of the help I received from the psychologist.

A battery of tests determined which areas of my brain were affected by the stroke and rehabilitation of those areas began. The areas affected were my reading (7th grade level), my spelling (6th grade level) and my math (8th grade level).

My verbal retention was zero. So I was very busy at home working on all my deficits, both physical and mental. Every day of my life, from the day I had my stroke to the day I die, I work on my deficits. Let me share with you now some of my observations which I hope will shed new light on the subject of stroke, things which may help the caregiver and the professional understand the stroke survivor.

The only way to describe my stroke is to say it was "a silent explosion" which took place in my brain. To this day I am still reaching out gathering bits and pieces of my brain trying to put it back together.

The first 72 hours after a stroke are the most critical. It is during that time that the stroke patient either will or will not respond to treatment. In my case, I overheard the doctor tell my wife about those first 72 hours, so I did not sleep. I was afraid that if I did I was going to die. If I fell asleep, I would never wake up. That time is also a period when the stroke survivor wants life surrounding him, especially at night. Being left alone at the hospital at night made me feel alone, forgotten and discarded.

Another effect of stroke is crying. It is a very normal part of stroke. Usually it begins to taper off about six to eight months after the stroke without ever completely stopping. In some cases, like my own, the crying never tapers off so I take medication to keep it under control most of the time.

Depression was and still is my biggest enemy as I continue to battle my stroke. This little enemy sits on my shoulder just waiting for the chance to attack. It has been five years since my stroke, so I have an advantage in my fight with depression. I know now when the depression is about to hit so I take steps to discourage it from taking over. In my case, depression usually hits me when I'm alone. The steps I take may be to change my environment or call someone on the telephone or maybe turn on the TV. My Black Labrador is also a great help in my fight against depression.

Fatigue, extreme fatigue, should be the middle name of most stroke survivors. Everything I do, from simple walking to simply trying to talk is fatiguing. Extreme fatigue from a stroke is a thousand times greater than the extreme fatigue a normal person feels after physical or mental activity. The stroke survivor has to try to pace himself so that his energy will last through the entire day's activities. Rest is the best medicine. The stroke survivor is not lazy. The brain has been violated and he is fighting back. That is a very fatiguing job.

Frustration is probably the thing most stroke survivors will deal with the rest of their lives. Trying to relearn the many things we learned as little children is frustrating. Not being able to relearn to do certain things ever again is frustrating. Everyday, from the day I had my stroke to the day I die, I must deal with frustration. It is something we must learn to live with.

Trust was a word which did not exist in my life during the early months of my stroke. I trusted no one. Not my doctor, my friends, loved ones, not even the one person I loved the most—my spouse. How could I trust anyone when I felt helpless, useless and a burden to everyone. It is the period in my life in which I lost all self-esteem, all pride and had no self-respect at all. Why? In my case, my spouse had to give me a bath, cut up my food, help put on my clothes, drive me places and wait on me hand and foot. Those things had not been done for me since I was a little child. I eventually got out of the distrust period but it takes a great deal of patience and love on the caregivers' part.

I hope caregivers and professionals now have a little better insight on why the stroke survivor can go in and out of periods of depression, have roller coaster emotions, become frustrated, angry, useless and feel unwanted. I, for one, am convinced that most stroke survivors should look into psychological help. I can't stress enough how important it was in speeding up my recovery.

Now what have I learned from my stroke and how do I live today? I have learned that everyday from now on is a rehabilitation day. I exercise all areas which were affected by the stroke, both physically and mentally. My motto is "use it or lose it."

I have also learned to love myself. The old Walt Collins is gone and I love the new me. Remember one thing, stroke survivors: We have been given a second chance at life. There have been many who never had that second chance.

The stroke had almost torn my marriage to shreds. But we weathered the storm, and now we have a stronger and closer relationship. I guess the best way to define this experience is by understanding and learning about "tough love."

Another thing I learned and keep in mind everyday is to never give up. Oh, how many times I wanted to give up. My doctor, my nurses and my occupational and physical therapists did not give up on me. My wife wouldn't give up on me, so I couldn't give up if I wanted to.

But there was one other source which was directly involved in my recovery. The Lord. Without the Lord in my life, my life today would be meaningless.

To close, I would like to leave you with four simple priorities which now guide my life day to day.

My God
My Family
My Work
My Health

from the Stroke Connection August 1988

The Task
of Caregiving

by Alice Beer, St. Paul, Minnesota

It's been more than 10 years now since my spouse suffered the first of two devastating strokes.

It's very difficult to enumerate the many changes that have happened to me in my daily living. I now must think for two people. I must protect and guide every action as a mother needs to watch over a child—an endless and exhausting responsibility. I wonder at times what it is that keeps me going from day to day. I am needed, and perhaps that's one reason.

I can't dwell too long on my losses because it saddens me and my morale sinks to low depths. But I do want to mention a few: I lost a companion, a protector, a driver, a financial advisor, a grocery shopper, a "fixit" man, a manager and most of all—I lost a caring, loving person—my husband. These are losses never to be regained.

In the meantime, I've had to "pull myself up by the boot straps." I have perhaps become stronger than I ever dreamed I might be, both emotionally and physically. I have few "free moments" but when I do, I *do* try to take care of myself. I must survive to fill this important, demanding role that I have chosen to accept. The days are never quite long enough. There are always more plans for errands, book work, etc. than can possibly be accomplished by one person. This is probably the most frustrating of all frustrations.

On the lighter and brighter side—it's through this new way of life that interesting channels have been opened to me. I have met wonderful people because of stroke. There are the volunteers from Catholic Charities who come to give respite care. They "sit" so that I can be away for a break. There are the nurses and the health aides, so kind to both of us! There are friends and relatives who relieve me so that I can go for an occasional massage, which is so therapeutic and does alleviate the arthritic aches and pains. There are neighbors who send in goodies so often; the passer-by who stops to chat while we're on our ramp for a little sunshine; the ladies of the Caregivers Support Group who understand and listen; those on the *Stroke Connection* committee who encouraged me to write this article; the girls in the church choir where I "sing my heart out" whenever I'm free to attend. All are my friends and help me so much more than they realize.

Never, before stroke, would I have felt equal to deliver a message before a group. Now I do; I have given presentations several times. I tell of my experiences in giving home care. I tell it "the way it is." So the task is not without its pluses even though it is never-ending. One does survive and somehow, one does grow!

from the Stroke Connection October 1981

The Triumphs of Stroke

by Chuck Steiger

There are common bonds of triumph shared by most persons who have been disabled by stroke. If you've had a stroke and are paralyzed on one side, and have achieved independence—to a reasonably high degree—you will know the joys and triumphs of hemiplegia that only others like you can or will ever experience.

Surely, it's hard to think of stroke in terms of joys and triumphs, but recall these benchmarks in your life:

Remember the day a comforting doctor told you that you had a stroke, that perhaps you'd almost died, but God wasn't ready for you yet, that you were doing just swell, and that you were going to take rehabilitation and keep on doing great? Does a mountain climber experience that exhilaration on reaching the summit?

Remember the fear in your heart when you began rehabilitation, and how it was dispelled by an encouraging therapist? He assured you of independence, didn't he? Could being the ringbearer at Prince Charles wedding be more thrilling? Or memorable?

Remember the first time you did with one hand what you'd done all your life with two, and were sure it couldn't be done, but you did it? Rolling a perfect game in bowling could not be more rewarding.

Remember the first time you dressed yourself with one hand, though you knew it couldn't be done? But you did it. Scaling Mt. McKinley could be no greater thrill.

Remember the first time therapists got you on your own two feet? You were frightened and wobbly, but your therapist assured you with the equivalent of a crane, derrick and hoist. And . . .there you were, upright. Even though three or four therapists and American Hoist and Derrick had been largely responsible, you felt pretty proud, and rightly so. Can a nonhemiplegic match the joy you experienced? Can a nonhemiplegic know the triumph you felt when loved ones lauded your progress?

This is not to advocate stroke as an avenue to joy, but if you've had a stroke and returned home, you're an Olympic gold medal winner.

Remember the first time you opened a milk carton with one hand? What a triumph! How about the first time you were free to wheel about in a wheelchair unrestrained? If you've recovered mobility, you'll recall the triumph of being free of that webbed belt and someone at your side. If you regained the ability to drive, you'll never forget your first "white knuckle" performance behind the wheel.

The process of recovering maximum independence from the disabilities of stroke has more than its fair share of ups and downs, ins and outs, trails and travails, triumphs and tragedies.

CVA—those mystical initials for Cerebral Vascular Accident—may have left us in varying hues of hemiplegia, but collectively we have had the fire, the fury and the determination that have brought us dividends without parallel in our struggle to return.

You aphasics will remember the first time you tried to talk and the words just wouldn't come out. And you'll never forget the first time the right words did come out. What a triumph!

You hemiplegics with field cuts will recall your distress when you tried to draw a straight line and couldn't, and when you discovered you were missing words on the left when trying to read, and you couldn't find things you know were there on the left side of your bedside table.

Those of you who enjoy the benefits of the Radio Talking Book and the National Library Service for the Blind and/or Physically Handicapped will recall the joy of realizing these offered you vast treasuries of books, magazines and publications, read aloud to you by experts.

The mileposts of stroke are too many to enumerate. Like the first time you put your socks on with one hand. The first time you opened a can with one hand. The first time you made a complete dinner with one hand. The first time you showered, bathed or otherwise performed personal grooming with one hand. The first time you cleaned house. And on and on and on. Each "first" was a milestone; each a triumph few can experience.

What's more, you've discovered you're not alone with your problems. You've discovered the benefits of sharing in a stroke club and coming to know fully that your problems are shared with others, and that through confidence and understanding, solutions can be found when you thought none existed.

Having been through rehabilitation programs, we have learned to adapt skills to disability, and vice versa.

The triumphs of stroke? The joys of stroke? Do strokes spawn triumphs and joys? No way.

But achieving independence after a stroke can and will produce some share of triumph and joy. Even though it may have to be shared with equal doses of tears and heartbreak.

from the Stroke Connection April 1983

To My Mother

by Stephanie Rasmussen DeWilkins, Palm Bay, Florida

Ten years ago, when I was away at college, my mother had a stroke. I really didn't know what one was and I was pretty removed from the full impact it had on her and the other members of my family. The stroke not only changed her, but me too.

I remember coming home from school the day she was to have surgery to remove the clot in her neck and I was scared that she was going to die. I made her promise me, before she went into surgery, that she wouldn't.

I realized then how much I had taken her for granted and I still think of how empty my life would be without her.

It's hard for me to put into words how I feel about my mother. She's always been there for me. But, someday she won't be, and I want her to know *now* how I feel.

> *I've never really thanked you*
> *For all the things you've done.*
> *You've cooked and cleaned and sewed and scrubbed,*
> *And I've kept you on the run.*
>
> *At times you really get angry,*
> *And I can be a witch,*
> *But Mom I want to tell you*
> *I don't ever want to switch.*
>
> *You know I love you Mom,*
> *Although we often fight.*
> *And I hope you don't feel too bad*
> *When I hate it when you're right!*
>
> *So Mom, this is just to tell you*
> *When all is said and done*
> *Everyone has a mother*
> *But you're the greatest one.*

from the Stroke Connection May 1984

Weird, Indeed

by John Steenerson, Minneapolis, Minnesota

Why is it,
no one can see.
This strange way,
I feel.
But then,
how can they see.
I can't even see myself,
weird.
Yes indeed,
very weird
I always feel like,
I am in the twilight zone.
And I don't know why.
Why does this stroke,
have to be so weird.
I just want everything
to be the same,
can't you see.
Will it never be the same?
It's got me feeling so weird.
My family,
they don't understand.
My friends,
they try to understand,
but they cannot understand
what they cannot see.
It can't be weird forever.
It just can't be.
I know it won't be.
How can it be.

from the Stroke Connection May/June 1988

What Should I Tell My Children about My Stroke?

by Marion Rasmussen, St. Paul, Minnesota

When does a stroke really start? What leads up to the acute stage or the onset? Could mine have been prevented? And what should I tell my children and their children about my stroke that would possibly influence their life styles so that they would be spared the agony of stroke? Perhaps if they chance to read this article, they might take heed. It is so easy to think that any misfortune happens to that "other guy" and not to ourselves. "Tain't necessarily so."

My father and his brother both died from heart disease at age 31. My husband's father died at age 49 from a coronary. My husband had a coronary at 43, another at age 60, even after a heart bypass. Two of my brothers have had coronaries and I had a stroke at 53 years of age. With that kind of family history, I feel that I am living on borrowed time. I feel lucky that I have lived past the age of 50 and that I have two daughters and three grandchildren.

I didn't realize until my children had children how much fathers mean to children. I missed a lot of life growing up without my father, who died when I was four years old. I remember that as a child I hated weekends, especially Sunday because I had no playmates because Sunday was the day fathers spent time with their children and family, going swimming, going on picnics or just for a drive in the country. I remember feeling envious and left out. I missed that special relationship that usually exists between daughters and fathers. I hope my daughters and my grandchildren will not be deprived of their loved ones prematurely because those loved ones failed to comply with good health-related rules.

My stroke was caused by a thrombus, which is a clot that forms in a cerebral artery, blocking the flow of blood to the brain. My stroke resulted in right-sided paralysis and aphasia, which is the loss or reduction in the ability to speak, read, write and comprehend the spoken word. Through therapy I have regained most of my independence. However, the principal problem of my stroke was the aphasia, one of the most frustrating and demeaning conditions I have ever experienced. That impairment, which took months with a speech therapist to correct, still plagues me to a very small degree.

In April of 1973, before my stroke, I sought a new internist who advised me to lose weight and go on a low-fat cholesterol-free regime because of my high blood pressure. I did so half-heartedly. I spent a busy summer that year, working on my masters degree, attending several refresher courses, developing an individualized study program for one of the courses I was teaching, getting my daughter ready for college and doing the household tasks that a "Supermom" usually did. I fell into bed at 10 p.m. exhausted. I had the world on a string and was enjoying every minute of my life, which was exciting and challenging. But that life changed overnight. Heredity, lack of dietary control and stress caught up with me and taught me some valuable lessons. The impact of my stroke still trickles down to our present daily life. My career as an instructor in medical records was at an end. In fact, my ability to work outside of my home was destroyed. My income had been meant to help educate my daughters. They now had to finance their own education. The week that I was discharged from the hospital, my husband was laid off from work and was not reemployed for five months. We lived frugally those five months. Ten years later, he also became permanently disabled as a result of heart surgery. The surgery left him with short-term memory loss. Our health-related problems have resulted in a cumulative loss of compensation over the years. Could this loss have been avoided? You bet!

The stress of stroke touches each member of the family. In my case, with one daughter away at college, the burden of housekeeping and transportation for me fell on the shoulders of my husband and my 16-year-old daughter, who was a high school junior with a part-time job. My older daughter cleaned the stables as her part-time job at college, getting up at 5 a.m. each morning.

I feel the greatest burden of stress on the family came from my aphasia. It was very difficult for us to conquer the frustration of my inability to communicate successfully. None of us plotted murder, but there were times...We still deal with some aspects of my aphasia, but we can now laugh at what we call my "stroke humor." We have developed little aids that smooth the friction caused by my aphasia.

My physical disability is still a nuisance, but I feel very fortunate to be as able as I am. I have no compaints—my husband does! He hates the housework that I am not able to do which he has to do.

Our lifestyle has been noticeably changed. Entertaining friends for dinner is just about out of the question for me unless one of my daughters helps me. If I could blindfold the guests or if I could let the house stay in its usual state of disorder, I would entertain with pleasure. I am not a prissy housewife, but I am uncomfortable if my home is untidy when expecting guests. My guests, for the most part, are my family. Even then, I plan ahead and pace myself. In fact, I try to pace myself in all of my endeavors so that I don't get over-tired.

So what should I tell my children about stroke? I failed miserably as a parent regarding my health. I did not lose weight; I did not follow a low-cholesterol, low-fat diet; I did not exercise; I did not reduce the stress in my life. I lived it up, burning the candle happily at both ends. I dared the fates. For some reason I thought I was exempt from misfortune. My biggest mistake.

What I want to tell my children and their children (and I hope everyone is listening)is:

- **Our family is at risk.** Take heed now before you end up like your parents, limping through the rest of your lives.
- Listen to your doctor and follow his advice about diet, exercise and reducing stress.
- Dare to be different from the rest of the world if your health would be in jeopardy by going along with the crowd.
- Start training your children early in life as far as the rules are concerned.

- Take your health seriously but don't become a hypochondriac.

- Take time **now** to enjoy your family and friends. Money is important but your health and family are far more important.

- Be happy and content. Don't ask for the moon. Strive to reach your goals but don't let the striving deprive you of your health, happiness and family.

- Laugh as much as you can. Humor got us through a lot of tight places.

- Balance your lives—some fun, some seriousness. Don't be a slave to tidiness. God and your friends won't mind the round corners in your house.

- Let God be your best friend. Have faith.

- Very important! **Nothing in the world—absolutely nothing—is worth having a stroke.**

I regret all the time I took from my family recovering from my stroke, time that could have been spent far more pleasurably. I regret missing the happy events we could have experienced together; the times that, because of my fatigue, I could not participate fully. I regret the times some member of the family needed me and I failed them because of my physical disability.

I hope my children will read this article and give pause to reflect on their life styles. Need I say more?

from the Stroke Connection May/June 1987

When Sudden Disability Occurs in Your Family

by Marion Rasmussen, St. Paul, Minnesota

Of course, you never think a serious illness or disability is going to happen to you or your family. Those things happen to the "other guy." I think none of us is prepared to deal with sudden illness or disability. But it does happen to you, just as it happened to me and my family 13 years ago.

We have lived through my stroke, grasping eagerly at every help. We've had good times and bad times. There were times when I wanted to run away, and I am sure there were times when my family wished the problems caused by my stroke would magically disappear. Many times I resented my family and they resented me for the problems accompanying my stroke. Many formerly close friends have disappeared, but new ones who are just as valuable have filled the void. For me, fatigue is a constant companion. For me and the members of my family, frustration still lurks in the background, waiting to threaten our composure when our defenses are down. But we have survived and we have survived more than just my stroke.

Since my stroke, we have survived the guilt of placing my mother-in-law in a nursing home and then seeing her through a leg amputation and finally a massive stroke which ended her life.

We have survived open-heart surgery for my husband with a consequential short-term memory loss and his forced early retirement.

We have survived my own mother's death, which was preceded by a two-year period of small strokes and accompanying mental deterioration, requiring 24-hour home-health attendants.

We have survived my husband's second heart attack, with catheterization performed the same day that my daughter gave birth to her second child, who was born with spina bifida.

We have survived all this and are grateful for what we have, and we are grateful for the problems we have rather than the problems many of our friends have. Our family situation is not unique. Many families are living with multiple-health problems, and disability is only one of the many setbacks and disappointments the family faces through life.

When a family is faced with sudden disability of one of its members, an array of emotions often overwhelms it—guilt, pity, resentment, sorrow, anger or frustration. Dealing with these varied emotions at a time of immense stress sometimes leaves you feeling absolutely helpless. Family members have their own needs and their own set of values, but in times of crises these values and needs run headlong into the needs of others, causing conflict. In my own case, when my mother and my mother-in-law were ill, I felt that some members of the family were not pulling their share of the weight. This situation happens in many families, and it often leads to anger, hard feelings, bitterness, frustration and resentment.

If relatives live out of town, there is still a feeling of resentment because they are missing the day-to-day action. Even if they come for a weekend, they cannot possibly know the constant stress of "living on the edge"—the edge of hope or despair. I have said jokingly that in my next life I want to live out of town, but out-of-town members have their own set of problems. They feel guilty because they are not at hand to give help. They are sad because they cannot be with their loved ones. And they may feel as though they are being left out, on the outside looking in. And there are some members who are too busy to help in any way whether they are in town or out of town, or they can't stand the smell of the hospital or nursing home. It's difficult not to resent those members. Many people do things they don't want to do but do anyway out of love or concern or pity for another human being.

The day my daughter went into labor with her second child, I was with my husband in another hospital waiting for him to undergo a heart catheterization. As soon as he left the room for the procedure, I called my daughter to see how she was doing. She had already delivered a baby boy. When she came to the phone she told me she had delivered a baby with spina bifida. "Mother," she asked, "what does that mean?" I explained as simply as I could and hung up. Then I sat alone in that hospital room and wept because I thought I could not face another tragic event. The pain of little Andrew's disability has not left me. I live with the pain of seeing my daughter and her husband coping with all the problems they face: 24-hour nursing care for Andrew; his tracheostomy; his being respirator-dependent; dealing with their 5-year-old daughter; coordinating schedules; both parents working full-time; no privacy; their incessant fatigue. I know by the hard edge of the brittleness in my daughter's voice, a hint of despair, when something is wrong—a breakdown in family communication, a nursing-care problem or a temporary, but life-threatening, illness of Andrew.

Andrew was in the hospital six months before he could come home. There is not much I can do except listen, babysit, try to understand, learn as much as I can about spina bifida and give as much comfort as I can. Their friends have drifted away; relatives have also drifted away. Is it too painful for them to see Andrew as disabled rather than "a little boy" whose parents need support? Again, we see how stressful disability is on all members of the family.

What can be done to help the family? In my case, I think if the hospital had used a team approach, some of our problems could have been solved much sooner with less stress. As it was, I turned to my physical and speech therapists. I used them as my "wailing wall" as I cried for help. There were no family counseling sessions where problems could be discussed and measures taken to rectify them. We simply floundered and eventually came to terms with my stroke. Close friends and relatives helped as much as they could, but the immediate family problems could have been addressed sooner and more effectively if we had had a structured program.

Another way to help a family is to encourage members to join a support group. A support group can give needed information, encouragement, answer questions and just give friendship when no one else seems to understand. There are support groups for the affected person, support groups for spouses, groups for caregivers, etc. One of the best moves I made after my stroke was to join (reluctantly at first) an aphasia support group. I felt that I had finally come home!

Professional counseling is another way to help. Counselors can give advice and teach coping skills. Perhaps, not all members are willing to seek counseling, but for those who are willing, it sometimes makes the difference between despair and hope.

For myself and family, my greatest resource of strength and comfort was from God. I am not one who kneels down everyday and prays and prays. I have a very personal relationship with God. I talk to and ask and thank God in simple everyday language. And I feel He walks beside me. This is the way I operate. Someone else may say I am foolish, that God doesn't work that way. Whatever way works for you is the best way. Wherever you find strength, hope and comfort, grab onto it, hold it, nurture it until your needs are fulfilled.

Living with a disability is a challenge. It is not easy. It is a bitter pill to swallow. But living with a disability also gives individuals an opportunity to learn about themselves and to find their strengths and weaknesses. It takes strength to face reality and live with it and make the best of it. The smile on Andrew's face makes all the efforts worthwhile.

from the Stroke Connection July 1987

Who Am I?

by Jeanette Weeks, Minneapolis, Minnesota

After visiting with a stroke survivor recently, I remembered that she kept stating, "I was really important before my stroke. I had an excellent position with my company that included many responsibilities." I have been trained as a peer counselor to inform her that we all are important, and she still is very important in spite of her stroke. It is very common for people to have their identity and worth tied to their role as a worker. The experience of surviving a stroke often damages a person's self-esteem and confidence.

I tried to reassure this young stroke survivor that her life is now different since her stroke. I told her that, before my stroke, I was a social worker and that my stroke has changed me and my lifestyle. However, I have continued to believe that I am important. As you know, stroke can strike anyone—whether you are a physician, a nurse, a teacher, psychologist, etc. I have dropped the idea that my identity is tied up with my role as a worker. I have been successful in finding valuable, worthwhile volunteer experiences outside of stroke that enable me to think of myself as being productive and worthy.

If you fall into that trap of holding onto your pre-stroke identity, please remember we are all important.

from the Stroke Connection May/June 1987

Why Psychotherapy?

by Jim Meier, Lake Elmo, Minnesota

The results of a stroke affect everyone, whether it be the survivor, a relative, a friend or a professional person. The major effort after a stroke is recovery. Therapeutic treatment must begin as soon as possible to increase the chances of correcting or improving what has been lost. To do that, physical, speech and occupational therapy should be administered to the survivor as soon as possible. The appropriate treatment continues until it is no longer necessary or feasible.

Psychotherapy is another very important sometimes necessary type of treatment that a survivor might need. That type of therapy could be required if a person is under stress, or if a person is hiding problems by using self-made "crutches," such as overeating, overwork, drugs, etc. The need for this type of therapy must not be overlooked by anyone.

Why is it important? Last fall, Walt Collins, a stroke survivor, was the keynote speaker at the annual Stroke Seminar at Courage Center and emphasized the importance of psychotherapy. The same topic was addressed in Walt's recent article in the *Stroke Connection*, titled, "The Silent Explosion" (see page 96). In both cases, Walt described what happened to him as "the parts of his mind were floating around in pieces, and he couldn't put them together." Walt spent several months under treatment with a psychologist reconstructing the results of the "explosion." Those sessions significantly helped Walt realign parts of his life to the point where both Walt and the therapist knew that he was "home."

The same type of "explosion" happened to me after I had my stroke in June 1983. During the months after the stroke, I was recovering from aphasia. The typical feelings that I had during that period were probably common to other survivors: I was bewildered, I realized what happened, I was angry and I became very depressed. It became clear that things were not working. Depression was obvious, stress and strain were apparent and it felt like something very bad was going to happen again. I needed help, and that help came from working with a psychologist.

From December 1983 through September 1984 I spent one hour, twice a month, with the therapist. The purpose was to regain self-confidence, overcome fear and start moving forward mentally again. I gained much from those sessions and was able to close some doors that were no longer needed. Instead, I found ways of seeing things more positively and knowing what my limitations were. A good example is the stress control exercise that I learned and now use. It's a six-step procedure that allows me to release mental pressure (sludge) by not even moving. It takes about 20 minutes of my time, it can be done any place and there is no cost. As one might say, it's like "cleaning the mental laundry."

If you feel that you are in a losing situation, or that you can't correct anything, or if anxiety and depression are common, talk to your doctor. Ask for help; don't be afraid. Maybe you can't eliminate physical or mental difficulties, but it does help you to understand and learn how to cope with them better. Speaking as a survivor, I assure you that psychotherapy works, and if it's needed, you should use it.

from Stroke Connection September/October 1986

You Don't Look Like You Had a Stroke

by Marion Rasmussen, St. Paul, Minnesota

"**Y**ou don't look like you've had a stroke!"

I have heard that statement time after time. And I wonder what I am supposed to look like after experiencing a stroke. Bedridden, in a wheelchair, arm in a sling, using a cane or a communication device? All of these signs may be indicative of stroke, but the active, involved stroke survivor, in spite of an aid such as a wheelchair or cane, belies the image of a useless, "throw-away" person.

It is estimated that 400,000 to 500,000 individuals experience stroke each year; about 230,000 survive. I am one of those survivors who doesn't look like I had a stroke. Through rehabilitation, drive, faith, luck and the support of my family, friends and a stroke club, I have returned (despite some deficits) to a life that is still full of challenge, full of promise, vital and worth living.

But I have not yet found a way to tell a person, in 25 words or less, what a stroke person goes through to get to where "you don't look like you had a stroke!"

How can I count up quickly the hours, days and months of practicing the once simple, automatic act of walking? Of trying to negotiate the stairs? The hours of exercise to strengthen my limbs? How can I count up the hours of occupational therapy relearning how to perform simple household tasks or tying my shoes? Or the hours my two daughters spent in reteaching me the skill of knitting and crocheting—the skill I taught them when they were barely old enough to hold a knitting needle or crochet hook? How can I count the hours I practiced writing, first with my unaffected hand and then with the

117

affected hand, while trying to remember how the letters of the alphabet were formed?

How can I tell about aphasia? What it means not to be able to understand the written or spoken word, much less speak the words? The agony of knowing what I wanted to say but not being able to verbalize? Or the agony of not being able to retrieve a word from that computer bank of words known as vocabulary?

How can I tell someone how it feels to not be able to add or subtract, to adjust a recipe or to modify a knitting pattern or balance a checkbook or compute taxes?

I sigh when I think about the emotional trauma of stroke—the feeling of abandonment, isolation, the big failures, small triumphs. I can remember the tears when I realized I could no longer "run with the pack" —golfing, playing bridge, driving and teaching. I remember the tears and resentment when I felt (mistakenly) my role as mother was being usurped by my mother, my daughters and my husband.

I can now do most of the things I did before my stroke. Those years after my stroke were "turmoil" years. The turmoil lessened as I grew stronger physically, mentally and emotionally through rehabilitation and learning to balance my assets and my deficits and learning to use alternative and creative methods of accomplishing tasks.

I, like many other stroke survivors, do not look like I had a stroke. But looking or not looking as if I had a stroke is not really important. What is important for me and others is that we are survivors, not victims; able though disabled; willing to work in spite of a handicap and part of a very caring section of the community. We have faced the changes in our lives, squared our shoulders and taken up active living.

The statement, "You don't look like you had a stroke," irritates me because it implies a negative image of a stroke person. When someone says that to me, I want to stand up, beat my fists on my chest Tarzan-like, raise a banner and proclaim, "I have overcome," but I usually reply with an inviting "ask me more" smile and say, "Oh, yes indeed I did." Just being there for all the world to see is visible proof that I belie the popular image of a stroke "victim!" Bury that image.